THE PROSTATE CANCER ESSENTIALS FOR SURVIVAL SERIES

RADIATION SAFETY AND PROSTATE CANCER: NEED YOU BE CONCERNED?

MICHAEL J. DATTOLI, MD

JOSEPH M. KAMINSKI, MD

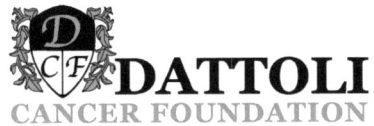

SARASOTA, FLORIDA

Prostate Cancer Essentials for Survival—Radiation Safety and Prostate Cancer: Need You Be Concerned?

Copyright © 2020 by Michael J. Dattoli, M.D. and Joseph M. Kaminski, M.D.

All rights reserved. No part of this work may be reproduced or transmitted in any form or by any means, electronic or mechanical, including photocopying or recording, or by any information storage or retrieval system, except as may be expressly permitted by the 1976 Copyright Act or in writing by the publisher.

ISBN-10: 1-9756815-6-8
ISBN-13: 978-1-9756-8156-2

Published by the Dattoli Cancer Foundation, Sarasota, FL
Book design and composition by Daniel van Loon, Batavia, IL

MEDICAL DISCLAIMER

This booklet is intended as a supplement but not as a substitute for the medical advice of a physician. It is imperative that you consult a qualified healthcare professional with regard to all matters relating to your health and particular situation. Neither the publisher nor the authors bear responsibility for any consequences due to the reader's decision to use any particular treatment, medication, dietary supplement or other healthcare practices discussed in this book.

DEDICATION

This booklet is dedicated to all those whose lives have been touched by prostate cancer, and to the patients and their families whom we are privileged to serve and educate as cancer care providers.

ACKNOWLEDGMENTS

We are deeply grateful to a number of people who have contributed to this booklet in a number of ways. Our thanks to Greg Lawrence, for his editorial efforts and to Ginya Carnahan, Chris Wells, Jone Fay, Donald Bryant, RT (R) (T) for their ongoing assistance.

We deeply appreciate all of those wonderful patients and family members who have contacted the Dattoli Cancer Foundation for counseling and guidance and in turn have given us their support and encouragement. It is your spirit and commitment in confronting this disease that inspires us all.

CONTENTS

INTRODUCTION

The Safety of Radiation in the Diagnosis and Treatment of Prostate Cancer 9

OVERVIEW—DIAGNOSIS AND TREATMENT RISKS

What is Radiation and How is it Used in Medicine? 13
What are CT Scans? 17
What is the Risk of Cancer with CT Scans? 18
What are MRI Scans? 25
What are Bone Scans and PET Scans? 26
What are the Risks of Immunodeficiency and Secondary Cancers after Radiotherapy? 27
What Are The Results of The Dattoli Combined Protocol? 30
Summary of the Dattoli 16-year Data 31

APPENDICES

A: Replacing LNT: The Integrated LNT-Hormesis Model 35
B: Deciding What is Best for You 39
C: Advanced Imaging and Treatment Planning at the Dattoli Cancer Center 41
D: Glossary of Medical Terms 45
E: The Warning Signs of Prostate Cancer 58

About the Authors 59
The Dattoli Cancer Foundation Mission 61
Order More Booklets in the Series 62

INTRODUCTION

THE SAFETY OF RADIATION IN THE DIAGNOSIS AND TREATMENT OF PROSTATE CANCER

The use of radiation in medicine has a long history to which scientists from diverse fields, such as physics, chemistry, engineering and medicine, have contributed over many decades. It was through the pioneering research of Madame Marie Curie working in France more than a century ago that the medical use of radiation, and X-rays in particular, first became a possibility. Our center is a part of that continuing history which allows us to provide our patients with the unique benefits of some of the most extraordinary advances of medical science in recent years.

Madame Curie's pioneering work on the theory of radioactivity and her role in the discoveries of polonium and radium took place at a time when no one even realized that radiation carried with it health risks, and therefore, no one took precautions to prevent overexposure to radiation. Madame Curie's death in 1934 was due to a form of aplastic anemia that had been caused by her many years of exposure to radioactive materials in the course of her research – she often carried test tubes of radium in her pockets. Ironically, her death occurred in the same year that her daughter, Irène Joliot-Curie, discovered what was called "induced" or "artificial" radioactivity, one of the early milestones in the field of nuclear medicine, which utilizes radionuclides (radioactive isotopes).

By 1946, radionuclides were being produced for medical use by the Oak Ridge National Laboratory. During the 1950s, the clinical use of nuclear medicine became widespread, as researchers increased our ability to detect and measure radioactivity and to use radionuclides to monitor biochemical processes. Many researchers in the U.S. and abroad worked to establish the efficacy, safety and therapeutic potential of this specialty. Over time, nuclear medicine has spawned a multifaceted industry that has progressed with countless remarkable technological innovations. The technical breakthroughs have been accompanied by the implementation of rigorous safety standards and strict regulatory oversight to ensure the safe use of radiation in medicine.

Radiation in a variety of forms now has multiple lifesaving applications in the diagnosis and treatment of many types of cancer, including prostate cancer. In a clinical setting like that of our center where we use the most sophisticated technologies currently available for the delivery of radiation, both the safety and efficacy of radiotherapy are augmented by patients coming to understand the basics of how radiation works and feeling confident about the standard of care that they receive.

As with all medical procedures, the safety of radiation is enhanced when patients are well informed about each particular test or course of therapy and there is a very clear line of communication between patients and the medical team. Patients should be informed as to what specific radiopharmaceutical or what kind of radiation will be used in their treatment or diagnostic procedure. And they should also be aware of exactly what safety precautions may be required.

All radioisotopes have a "half-life," which is how long the isotope takes to decay and become inert. Some patients may continue to emit detectable levels of radiation for periods of time after undergoing certain procedures or treatments. In those cases, precautions are taken. For example, some men may be advised to temporarily avoid prolonged exposure to young children, as is the case for prostate cancer patients who undergo brachytherapy, a mainstream procedure we offer that involves the implantation of radioactive seeds.

Patients who undergo certain nuclear medicine imaging procedures may require special preparation beforehand. For example, patients may need to stop taking some medications or follow certain dietary guidelines. At our center, the Dattoli team provides advice about exactly what preparation may be required of patients prior to a particular test or procedure in order to ensure their safety.

Our current protocols for Dynamic Adaptive Radiotherapy (DART), which is often combined with brachytherapy, utilize the latest cutting edge technologies for the diagnosis and treatment of prostate cancer. We have multiple, state-of-the-art systems in place to safeguard the patients under our care, as well as the doctors, nurses, technicians and support staff who comprise the Dattoli team. We are ever vigilant in this regard and we do far more than is mandated by federal and state oversight regulations to ensure the safety of our patients. This standard of care has been achieved thanks in part to the breathtaking progress in recent decades with both advanced imaging modalities and radiation delivery systems.

Our new technologies are making diagnosis, management, and treatment of prostate cancer and other diseases more sensitive, more specific, more effective and ultimately safer. With diagnostic imaging, we have seen a growing popularity of fusing modalities, such as combining the metabolic imaging of positron emissions tomography (PET), computed tomography (CT) scans and magnetic resonance imaging (MRI) scans. We are also taking advantage of the new role of therapeutic radiopharmaceuticals and contrast agents that use molecular targeting as a method of prostate cancer detection and localization, which can be either organ or tissue specific.

A radiopharmaceutical can be used for diagnostics or therapeutics, and can be administered to patients by injection, by swallowing or by inhalation. Once it has been administered, the chemical moves through the body to the specific organ or tissue to which it is attracted, before being metabolized and excreted from the body. As the chemical moves through the body, external devices can be utilized to detect the radiation it emits, which is used to generate computer images of the areas of interest and thereby locate cancerous lesions. Because the targeted radiation only travels a short distance, damage to healthy neighboring tissue or organs is minimized. These tests can be performed on an outpatient basis and most patients can go home after the procedure.

The purpose of this booklet is to enable patients to make informed decisions and enjoy peace of mind about their own choices with regard to both diagnostic laboratory tests and treatment procedures that utilize various forms of radiation. Many of our observations regarding the safety of diagnostic imaging and radiotherapy as they pertain to prostate cancer are also applicable to other cancers and diseases.

In our practice, the bottom line is that each diagnostic examination and each therapeutic procedure is conducted so the radiation dose to the patient is the lowest necessary to achieve our clinical aims. We share our patients' concerns about safety in part because we find ourselves working in close proximity to radiation sources each day. Yet we know that our exposure as well as that of our patients is well within safe limits.

We also know that the news media frequently misinforms the public about the risks of potential side effects from undergoing various procedures that utilize radiation, including radiological lab tests such as CT scans. Hopefully, this booklet can help dispel some of the alarmist myths that continue to circulate on the Internet and elsewhere. This is not to say there are no risks involved with the numerous applications of nuclear medicine and radiotherapy; but the evidence-based data from many published studies demonstrates that the immense benefits for patients greatly outweigh the risks of any harm, including possible radiation-induced side effects such as secondary cancers, which will be discussed in the pages ahead.

Prostate cancer is one of the most controversial fields of medicine, and physicians continue to disagree about which treatment options offer the greatest chance for cure with the least danger of side effects. We encourage patients to become informed, to ask questions and to be proactive – to demand the highest standard of care. In the end, whatever you decide as you consult with your physician with regard to diagnostic testing and treatment, you should feel confident at the end of the day that you have made the right choices for yourself based on your own particular needs and individual case.

OVERVIEW

DIAGNOSIS AND TREATMENT RISKS

What is Radiation and How is it Used in Medicine?

Radiation is a natural part of our daily lives and plays an essential role in the evolution of life on earth. X-ray radiation is a form of energy like visible light or radio waves. We are exposed to radiation from cosmic rays in our environment, from earth and soil, and from food and drink that may contain trace amounts of radioactivity. Every year all of us are exposed to this natural radiation as well as radiation from many other sources, including household smoke detectors, LCD televisions and computer displays. Air travel increases exposure to cosmic radiation due to the fact that there is less atmospheric shielding at higher altitudes. Even the human body naturally contains small amounts of radioactivity in the form of isotopes such as radium, potassium, and cesium.

Radiation is called "ionizing radiation" when it is strong enough to break molecular bonds either directly or indirectly, freeing electrons from atoms or molecules. These bonds can be broken in our DNA, the so-called building blocks of life. Ionizing radiation includes, X-rays, gamma rays, cosmic rays, high frequency ultraviolent light, and various atomic and subatomic particles, all of which can cause changes in the human body. Typical ionizing subatomic particles from radioactivity or radioactive decay include alpha and beta particles and neutrons. Low-energy radiation is called "non-ionizing radiation." This type of radiation includes visible light, sound waves, infrared waves, radio waves, and microwaves. Non-ionizing radiation does not possess enough photon energy (energy per quantum) to ionize molecules or atoms—that is, to remove an electron from a molecule or an atom.

The contention by some researchers that the low-dose ionizing radiation used in various forms in certain medical procedures may be carcinogenic has been controversial over the past two decades. The number of medical tests that utilize ionizing radiation has been increasing over the years. The United Nations Scientific Committee on Effects of Atomic Radiation has estimated that almost 3.6 billion X-ray examinations are now being performed worldwide every year. Researchers disagree about the small risk that is present when radiation is used for diagnosis and treatment, though it now appears that low-dose optimizing radiation poses even less of a health risk than previously believed.

The X-rays generated by machines that enable us to see inside the human body involve radiation exposure in addition to that from the ionizing radiation in the environment. The risk from exposure varies considerably depending on the energy and intensity of the X-ray radiation generated by a machine, and depending on the age and the sex of the person undergoing a medical imaging test, as well as the part of the body exposed and other factors such as the person's family history of cancer.

Ionizing radiation has been shown to be harmful in high doses. But it is not certain if there is significant harm from the much smaller doses of ionizing radiation that are used in diagnostic medical imaging. It is important to understand that the risk of radiation causing harm will vary depending upon its dose. However, it has been shown that risk varies for different groups of people. For the elderly, the risk is relatively small. For children and young females, the risk is slightly higher. Many researchers also believe that radiation risk is additive or cumulative, which means the more times a person has a test that utilizes ionizing radiation, the higher the risk. However, it should be noted again that as long as a person benefits from the test, many of which are potentially life-saving, those benefits will most likely far outweigh the risks.

Radioactive substances (radiopharmaceuticals) used for medical imaging are administered in very small amounts. Because researchers have studied the amount of radiopharmaceuticals that are needed for each test, the radiation dose to the patient can be minimized. Health problems that arise from the use of ionizing radiation in medical imaging are actually rare. However, some problems are sometimes reported and gain attention in the media, and they may seem to be more common than they actually are.

When directed at the body, X-rays penetrate tissue and are gradually absorbed. Some of the radiation is absorbed by cells and can damage the DNA that normally allows cells to function and reproduce. Cancer cells are somewhat more sensitive to radiation than are healthy cells, and therefore, the radiation used to destroy cancer cells is less likely to damage normal tissues, which are more resilient. However, this difference in sensitivity is generally small and the dose of radiation required to destroy prostate cancer cells is high enough that there is some risk of damage to healthy tissue in the nearby rectum or bladder. The strategy with radiotherapy over the years has been to deliver higher and higher doses more and more accurately to the targeted cancer, while sparing healthy adjacent tissue in order to avoid rectal and urinary complications.

Radiation is often measured by a unit called the Gray (Gy), which is roughly analogous to a Watt of light. Radiotherapists frequently describe radiation dose rates in terms of centigray (cGy), or 100 Gray (what used to be called a "rad"). Because radiation has different effects depending on the sensitivity of tissue it interacts with, different dose descriptors have been developed. Radiation dose is often described using the quantity known as "effective dose," which is measured in millisievert (mSv). This is essentially a tissue-weighted sum of the equivalent doses in all specified tissues and organs of the human body. Previously, units of measurement for radiation included the Curie (Ci), the radiation absorbed dose or RAD, and the Röntgen equivalent man (REM). The Gray and Sievert have now replaced the RAD and REM, respectively.

The effective dose represents the whole body dose that would give the same cancer risk as caused by the doses imparted to different organs in a specific part of the body. Effective dose offers a way to compare in approximate terms the relative risk between different radiation procedures. The effective dose quantitatively accounts for the relative sensitivities of the different tissues exposed, thus allowing for quantification of risk and comparison to sources of exposure such as natural background radiation and radiographic medical procedures like X-rays.

As mentioned, different kinds of imaging exams impart different amounts of radiation. The most common X-ray examination is the conventional chest X-ray. The X-ray imaging procedure imparts an average effective dose of approximately 0.02 mSv. In the comparative context of the radiation we are exposed to from natural sources, this is a relatively low dose. The average radiation dose from naturally occurring radioactive sources and cosmic radiation from outer space is about 2.4 mSv per year as a global average, which is slightly less than 80% of the total average dose received by humans. The rest of the dose that we are exposed to comes from artificial sources, including medical radiation at slightly less than 20% of the total average dose, while 40% is due to nuclear weapons testing fall-out, occupational exposure, nuclear power plant discharges and radiation from the Chernobyl accident.

The natural background doses vary around the country. People in the higher elevations of Colorado and New Mexico receive about 1.5 mSv more per year than people living in coastal areas near sea level. There are some geographical areas where people are exposed to as much as 10 mSv per year. The additional dose from exposure to cosmic rays during a round-trip flight from New York to Los Angeles is approximately 0.03 mSv. Altitude is a significant factor with cosmic rays, but the largest source of background radiation comes from radon gas in homes, which is about 2 mSv per year. Like other sources of background radiation, exposure to radon varies widely around the country.

To put it in simple terms, the radiation exposure from one chest X-ray is roughly equivalent to the level of radiation exposure we experience from the natural background of our environment in about 10 days.

With nuclear medicine scans, various radionuclides are combined with other chemical compounds to form the radiopharmaceuticals that are widely used in this field. When administered to patients, these radiopharmaceuticals can target specific organs and cellular receptors and selectively bind to them. As mentioned, external detecting devices are used to capture the radiation emitted from the radiopharmaceutical as it travels through the body and this information is used to generate images. Diagnosis is based on the way the body reacts to these substances in a healthy state versus the way it reacts when disease is present.

The radionuclide used is usually bound to a specific "tracer" that is known to act in a particular way in the body. When cancer is present in the body, the tracer may be distributed in a different way than when no cancer is present. Increased physiological function that may occur as a result of disease or injury usually results in an increased concentration of the tracer, which can often be detected as a "hot spot." Sometimes the disease leads to exclusion of the tracer and a "cold spot" may be detected. A large variety of tracer complexes are used in nuclear medicine to visualize the different organs and tissues in the body.

Nuclear medicine procedures are among the safest diagnostic imaging exams available; the amount of radiation received from a nuclear medicine scan is comparable to that of many diagnostic X-ray and CT procedures. The main difference between nuclear medicine diagnostic tests and other imaging modalities is that nuclear imaging techniques show the physiological function of the organ or tissue that is being investigated, while more traditional imaging techniques such as CT scans and MRI scans show only the anatomy or structure of the organs and tissue. The incredible specificity that we now have with this growing arsenal of imaging modalities has greatly improved the efficacy of advanced radiotherapy, such as DART in treating even high-risk and more advanced prostate cancers.

Since the 1950s, radiation therapy (RT) in various forms has been a common technique used for the treatment of many kinds of cancers. It is a standard treatment for prostate cancer that is clinically confined to the prostate gland and surrounding tissues (Stages T1, T2, and T3). At our center, we often combine the most advanced techniques of external radiation (DART) with radioactive implants (brachytherapy). External radiation may be prescribed for patients with prostate cancer that has spread to the pelvic and abdominal lymph nodes. Patients with advanced prostate cancer (metastatic disease) may also be treated with external radiation as a palliative (non-curative) therapy to reduce the size of the tumor and alleviate symptoms.

Patients with a limited number of metastases (cancer that has spread to a few sites—lymph nodes and/or bones) have what is known as Oligometastatic disease, and these patients may benefit from treatment with DART in order to take these areas of disease out of the equation. As noted, our ability to visualize these areas so we can aim at them with greater accuracy has dramatically improved in recent years. We believe that we are giving these men with aggressive disease an additional lease on life and allowing them to preserve their quality of life as long as possible.

What are CT Scans?

The CT scan (also called CAT scan) uses computer tomography to produce a 3-dimensional image of the prostate and surrounding organs. CT scans rely on computer-reconstructed X-rays to give a cross-sectional view of the body. A CT scan through the pelvis reveals the distinct outline of the prostate.

CT scans can identify prostate enlargement and show the size and shape of the gland, but it is not as effective for assessing the extent of cancer or visualizing cancer within the gland itself. While CT scans provide less defined images of the outer prostatic contour and internal architecture, CT images do accurately delineate the spatial relationship between the prostate, rectum and pubic bones. More contemporary spiral or helical CT scans provide greater resolution while taking less time to acquire the information, and thus, far less radiation exposure. The latest CT software enables full 3-dimensional reconstruction.

The arm of the CT scanner directs pinpoint-thin X-ray beams through the portions of the body under examination as it rapidly passes over the patient. Each pass of the CT scanner provides a cross-section of the body's internal structures, and as many as eight scans per centimeter are taken.

The data is fed into a computer, which converts the information into a three-dimensional image. The image gives a more precise and accurate picture of the internal organs than the flat view provided by conventional X-rays, since they superimpose overlapping organs and can only dimly represent the soft tissues of the body.

The main advantages of the CT scan over the other modalities are that CT offers a finer delineation of sources and more accurate imaging of the pubic bones. In addition, the CT requires less patient preparation and is less operator-dependent than transrectal ultrasound (TRUS), which does not use ionizing radiation. The CT scan is widely used for post-implant dosimetry and quality control with brachytherapy. The primary disadvantage of CT-based seed implants is the lack of real time imaging. While CT scans provide less defined images of the outer prostatic contour and internal architecture, CT images do accurately delineate the spatial relationship between the prostate, rectum and pubic bones.

More contemporary spiral or helical CT scans provide greater resolution while taking less time to acquire the information. At our institution, a GE High Speed Helical CT Scanner captures high resolution, 3-dimensional images of the prostate, seminal vesicles, bladder, urethra and rectum, which are required to accurately design individual treatment plans. This scanner is also equipped to perform QCT Bone Density evaluations for patients undergoing hormone therapy (androgen deprivation therapy, or ADT) as part of their treatment.

A University of Washington study compared TRUS and CT volumes drawn independently by three observers (Badiozamani, Wallner and Blasko). They reported the imaging modalities were consistent in measuring anterior-posterior, lateral and cranial-caudal dimensions (Badiozamani et al, Comparability of CT-based and TRUS-based prostate volumes. Int J Radiat Oncol Bioi Phys. 1999 Jan 15;43 (2):375-8). The significance of this finding is that CT and TRUS images are actually in close correspondence in determining pre-treatment volumes. When interpreted correctly, the CT and TRUS volumes are virtually interchangeable.

Today the CT scan is often combined or fused with other sophisticated imaging and diagnostic modalities, such as MRI scans, PET scans, and a number of dynamic contrast agents, including ultrasmall superparamagnetic iron oxide (USPIO). These fused imaging modalities represent the state of the art and have greatly enhanced our ability to safely diagnose and treat prostate cancer and many other diseases.

What is the Risk of Cancer with CT Scans?

There are a number of doctors who have issued warnings about patients undergoing CT scans regularly during routine checkups, suggesting that a CT scan is not worth the risk of even such a small amount radiation exposure because it will lead to an increased risk of leukemia or other cancers. Some critics also suggest that CT scans are done primarily to increase financial revenues rather than benefit patients. We believe the case against CT scans is a myth that does not hold up to rigorous analysis of the evidence-based data.

What is the rationalization for CT scans causing cancer? According to this argument, the ionizing radiation of CT scans may hit a DNA strand and cause it to mutate and become cancerous. There is also a secondary phenomenon involving oxygen molecules. What happens is the incident radiation particle comes in as a photon, and it hits the oxygen molecules and scatters the oxygen into free radicals, which in turn also hit DNA strands and can break those bonds or alter them.

Does this process actually cause damage to cells? Various media accounts have suggested that it does and have discouraged people from having CT scans, in much the same way the media has tried to discourage men from having PSA tests and women from having mammograms. We think this may be part of the reason we are seeing so many men with advanced prostate cancer, because many men are now avoiding PSA testing. Men are often reticent to talk about their health and their private parts, erectile dysfunction and so on. So when they are mistakenly informed that they don't need PSA testing anymore, that the test will not benefit them, they often put off being tested until symptoms of the disease can no longer be ignored, giving prostate cancer the chance to become advanced and be spread throughout the body.

It may be telling to compare some of the healthcare recommendations that we read in the media with the kind of healthcare that our U.S. presidents typically receive and the kinds of routine diagnostic testing they undergo. The former presidents appear to be blessed with longevity. Jimmy Carter is 95 years old and only recently facing a serious challenge with cancer. Reagan was 93 and suffered from Alzheimer's when he passed away. He also had colorectal cancer that was picked up early through diagnostic testing. Likewise, Gerald Ford lived into his nineties. Most of our modern presidents have long lifespans despite the stresses they endure. One of the reasons for their longevity might well be the annual "executive physicals" that they receive.

The Mayo Clinic is famous for conducting executive physicals, which they offer to heads of state and corporations. Our center also offers this kind of extensive physical on an annual basis to our patients. We don't push that kind of physical examination on our patients, but we do offer it to them. And we also listen to the media and try to address what may be concerns, which is one reason that we obtained at great expense the latest generation of CT scanner technology. Our machine gives very low radiation exposure, with extremely high resolution. It delivers only 1 mSv (millisievert) of exposure to the body, which is very low compared to even the previous generation of CT scanning machines, which are still widely in use at other institutions and register about 5 mSv of radiation exposure.

The reality is that alarmist studies on CT scanning have been basing the data on what is called the "linear no-threshold model," or LNT, which is now widely considered obsolete and erroneous. The linear no-threshold model has been used since the 1970s in radiation protection to quantify radiation exposure and set regulatory limits. The model assumes that the long-term, biological damage and cancer risk caused by ionizing radiation is directly proportional to the dose. The risk of low doses was extrapolated from the risk calculated at higher doses. According to this model, radiation is always deemed to be harmful with no safety threshold, that is, no mater how low the dose of radiation. The additive effect of radiation exposure over time with this model would mean that a series of very small exposures would have the same effect as one larger exposure. That kind of reasoning is more and more being challenged these days.

Before he joined the Dattoli team, Dr. Joseph Kaminski contributed to a 2009 article that called into question the basic premises of the LNT model for determining the risk of low-dose radiation exposure (Tubiana M, Feinendegen LE, Yang C, Kaminski JM. The linear no-threshold relationship is inconsistent with radiation biologic and experimental data, Radiology. 2009 Apr; 251(1):13-22. doi: 10.1148/radiol.2511080671).

That article concluded, "It is unethical to fuel anxiety with debatable hypotheses…A balance should be made between the risk, if any, of an X-ray examination and the medical information it provides…LNT was a useful model half a century ago. But current radiation protection concepts should be based on facts and on concepts consistent with current scientific results and not on opinions. Preconceived concepts impede progress; in the case of the LNT model, they have resulted in substantial medical, economic, and other societal harm."

The findings of that study and others led the United Nations Scientific Committee on the Effects of Atomic Radiation (UNSCEAR) to issue new policy recommendations in 2014 that departed from the LNT model for exposure below background levels of radiation. The UNSCEAR report to the U.N. General Assembly stated that "the Scientific Committee does not recommend multiplying very low doses by large numbers of individuals to estimate numbers of radiation-induced health effects within a population exposed to incremental doses at levels equivalent to or lower than natural background levels." Dr. Kaminski published a more recent study on this subject, which is included in Appendix A of this booklet (Kaminski CY, Replacing LNT: The Integrated LNT-Hormesis Model, Dose-Response, 2020, April-June).

A 2016 paper from the Fox Chase Cancer Center provides an accurate assessment on current policies regarding safety regulations and low dose ionizing radiation. The abstract reads in part:

There is considerable disagreement in the scientific community regarding the carcinogenicity of low-dose radiation (LDR), with publications supporting opposing points of view. However, major flaws have been identified in many of the publications claiming increased cancer risk from LDR. The data generally recognized as the most important for assessing radiation effects in humans, the atomic bomb survivor data, are often cited to raise LDR cancer concerns. However, these data no longer support the linear no-threshold (LNT) model after the 2012 update but are consistent with radiation hormesis" (Doss, M., "Future Radiation Protection Regulations," Health Phys. 2016 Mar;110(3):274-5).

The discredited LNT model is what leads some researchers even today to continue making false assertion that CT scans expose patients to enough radiation to cause cancers. The state-of-the-art CT technology at our institution is constantly upgraded to alleviate patient concerns about CT scanning, however misplaced those concerns may have been because of media-driven distortions.

With that said, through the years we have had many patients with early stage lung cancers whose lives were saved thanks to early detection. Those would have been advanced cancers had we not diagnosed them early with CT scans. We have also seen similar early detection with CT scanning save the lives of patients with pancreatic and renal cancers, and those patients would have surely died were it not for early diagnosis and treatment. And we have had patients with a host of other conditions like abdominal aneurysm that would have become life-threatening if we had not detected them with CT scans.

At our facility patients pay about $430 out of pocket for CT scans with our advanced machine. That's about the copay they would have to pay if they went elsewhere and had CT scans on the older, less expensive scanners. So we are certainly not having patients undergo CT scans in order to generate a revenue stream, given that our expensive machine is not reimbursed any more than the other less expensive CT scanners that most other institutions utilize. We perform these scans only for the benefit of our patients.

When we find patients who have advanced prostate cancer, we perform advanced imaging including CT scanning to detect lymph node involvement. We know exactly where to look and we know if those lymph nodes are enlarged, regressed, if they've come back, and so forth. That is all very important data that allows us to appropriately treat patients and in many cases save their lives.

One lab test that men receive with their executive physicals when they come to us each year is called a QCT-BMD bone density exam. This is an elaborate DEXA type scan which women get starting at age fifty, sometimes sooner. It is usually given when they are post-menopausal. We use this test in part because men actually have increased risk for osteoporosis and osteopenia much like women do. Interestingly when men develop hip fractures, for example, they have a two-fold risk for that becoming a fatal injury. We often see men who are sedentary, who smoke cigarettes, who drink alcohol, who have a thyroid disorder or chronic GI distress, or undergo prolonged hormonal therapy, experience bone mineral decline like women do.

What we do differently at our center is this. Women undergo what is called a DEXA scan. That scan is an excellent technique and a standard in endocrinology. Other institutions such as the National Osteoporosis Foundation suggest that all men starting at age fifty should be tested. We take this DEXA scan a step further. When a typical DEXA scan is done, we are looking at a cortical bone. That is the outside of the bone that you may think of when you see images of the skeleton. However, what the DEXA scan can't measure is the inside of the bone, that is, the mushy, interior part of the bone where the bone marrow is.

With our scanner, we can measure that interior and it's actually a forecast of what is going to be seen in the near future in terms of bone health or deterioration. In other words, the extra-skeletal bone is what it is; however, the marrow inside of the bone is a forecast of what the future of the bone will be. So we look at both the inside and outside and treat a patient accordingly, because if the trabecular marrow is not healthy, that predicts that the outer bone is also going to be unhealthy in the future.

All of this is expensive. A typical Dexa scanner may cost $50,000, but in order to do a QCT-BMD as well, we need an advanced CT scanner and the software program, which is hundreds of thousands of dollars. This is typically another part of the executive physical done at our institution when men choose to have it done. Again, this is an option for them, and we aren't trying to push it on our patients. But many of our men are pretty savvy and already having annual executive physicals. Many were or are among the best and brightest of CEOs and other leading professionals in their fields, and they are accustomed to having this standard of care each year and simply want to have the scan done.

As mentioned, with our CT scanner, patients receive 1.0 mSv of radiation. If you take a flight from New York to London, you are exposed to more radiation in your body than a CT scan. So if you do a lot of traveling, you are essentially getting the equivalent of multiple CT scans. And what about the pilots? What about the flight crew? In fact, because of their exposure to cosmic rays at high altitudes, they are exposed to a higher radiation dose than nuclear power plant workers. Are pilots and flight crews and their unions concerned about their safety? Are they being tested for leukemias and other potential secondary malignancies? No, they are not, because the risk is negligible or simply nonexistent.

It would be absurd for us to warn pilots about a danger that in reality does not exist. If we had ever heard about pilots or flight attendants being diagnosed with cancer at an alarming rate, we would know that by now. Obviously, commercial airplanes and their crews have been around quite a long time.

Radiologists are working with ionizing radiation all the time. What about radiation technologists? What about cardiologists? What about the physicians at our center? We are exposed to relatively high doses by just handling the radioactive seeds that we use for brachytherapy. We receive far more radiation than a CT scan imparts, and we have had that kind of exposure over many years without being at risk for radiation-induced cancers.

The people who were exposed to the atomic bomb at Hiroshima and Nagasaki have been well tracked over the years since the time of the bombing. There was a group around the perimeter that did get very high, toxic doses and died from radiation poisoning and toxicity. But many others just outside the perimeter didn't. What they were subject to and harmed by was fire, not radiation. They were breathing contaminated air and eating contaminated food and they may have had an increase in carcinogenic levels, as did victims of the Holocaust, from the poor nutrition and stress they lived in. They had a higher risk, but they didn't suffer from any radiation poisoning.

Likewise, the 9/11 victims who were in close proximity of that disaster have also been tracked. Many of them have developed cancers in the years since. But they were not radiated; they were simply in harm's way and breathed in toxic fumes. So people living in that general vicinity of downtown New York City are being followed, and they have had an increase of developing malignancies, especially firefighters, compared to the rest of the population at large, not because of radiation but because of other risk factors, like stress, bad air, toxic fumes.

Chernobyl is another illustrative case. There were people who were in the perimeter and about two dozen people did die from radiation poisoning. But outside of that pool of patients, the number of radiation casualties was extremely low. About 200,000 people were evacuated from that catastrophe and never came back, even though it's a very popular destination today for tourists. There were as many as 1,250 suicides because of the radiation scare after the event, with many people fearing that they were doomed to develop cancer after exposure. 200,000 women had abortions after Chernobyl because of that kind of psychological terror.

Indeed, the risk of low-level radiation was far more psychological than physiological. A 2005 study reported that "the mental health impact of Chernobyl is the largest public health problem unleashed by the accident to date" (Andrew C. Revkin, "Nuclear Risk and Fear, from Hiroshima to Fukushima," *New York Times*, March 10, 2012) In fact, there was a small cancer risk for people who were close to the perimeter at Chernobyl, but the risk was thyroid cancer, which is very curable. So we believe only much greater doses can cause cancers, because very high doses of radiation can overwhelm what is known as "natural DNA repair."

We are all walking, breathing DNA repair machines. We have discussed ionizing radiation and oxygen. All living organisms have been subject to DNA radicals being shot out from oxygen and have learned to repair the damage. There are repair mechanisms of action in the body that actually appear to reduce the rate of cancer. This has been going on since the first appearance of organic molecules. We believe the process of DNA repair has actually perfected itself to the point where people who have been subjected to cumulative low doses of radiation, like those living at high altitudes, have a very low incidence of cancer.

The longest-living people in the world are those who live in the Himalayas and they have a lower risk of developing cancers than those of us living at lower altitudes – as much as 30% lower risk. So DNA repair suggests that low dose radiation may actually be good for you. This theory is known as radiation hormesis. It is predicated on the protective ways that our bodies cope with radiation and repair damage, taking care of mutant cells and not allowing their progression.

Proponents of hormesis argue that low doses of ionizing radiation within or slightly above natural background levels are beneficial, because the radiation stimulates the activation of DNA repair mechanisms that protect us against cancer. According to this theory, DNA repair mechanisms are effective enough to reverse the detrimental effects of low-dose ionizing radiation. It's a repair mechanism that has been in place since the beginning of life and it's only gotten better over time as our bodies have adapted. It's an evolutionary adaptation that protects humans and all other species.

Given the available evidence and most recent studies, we believe radiation is certainly not toxic in low doses like that generated with CT scans. It is also telling perhaps that most healing springs have radiation in their waters. These springs probably expose us to the radiation of about ten CT scans done by the older generation of scanners without increased risk of cancer.

What are MRI Scans?

Magnetic resonance imaging (MRI) is an imaging technique that generates a magnetic field, which harmlessly reacts with the tissues of the body to produce a distinct and complex image of internal organs. MRI scans utilize a radiopharmaceutical contrast agent to enhance imaging, which is known as Dynamic Contrast Enhanced MRI (DCE-MRI).

The endorectal MRI is much like an ultrasound probe in that it is placed in the rectum and allows us to image the prostate very closely. It is a very detailed test for looking at the capsule of the prostate and determining whether or not there is cancer that has extended outside of the prostate capsule. Magnetic resonance spectroscopic imaging (MRSI) is a scanning method that provides spectroscopic information in addition to the image that is generated by MRI alone. The Dynamic Contrast Enhanced MRI is proving to be superior to the spectroscopic MRI as the true gold standard among the imaging modalities known as Multiparametric MRI.

At our institution, most patients undergo an MRI (preferably Dynamic Contrast Enhanced MRI) in addition to 3D Color-Flow Power Doppler Ultrasound (which utilizes only sound waves) and 2.0 mm fine section helical CT prior to prostate brachytherapy and/or DART. The only reason a patient wouldn't have an MRI is if his insurance company doesn't cover it and the patient can't afford the test, as it is expensive. The cost of a diagnostic pelvic MRI can be two to three times higher than the cost for a TRUS or CT. Setting aside cost considerations, the art of advanced radiation planning and design depends in large part on optimal integration of these complementary imaging modalities.

As noted, any risk involved with these imaging techniques is far outweighed by the benefits. Taken together, all of these tests enable us to accurately visualize various physical aspects of the prostate, such as its size, shape and contour. The tests also provide us with detailed information about the volume and location of the tumor sites. With this information, we are able to determine the optimal protocol for treating the disease, deriving in advance a unique treatment blueprint for each individual patient.

What are Bone Scans and PET Scans?

A bone scan is an imaging technique used to detect bone metastases, which appear as "hot spots" on film. It is far more sensitive than conventional X-rays. The typical bone scan procedure is performed by injecting a small amount of radioactive dye called technetium into the patient's bloodstream. A special camera is then used to photograph the skeleton, and any irritation of the bone will show up as a spot on the image. The amount of radiation exposure with this test is very low, comparable to CT scans.

If a patient's PSA is greater than 10, or if the Gleason score is greater than or equal to 7, we usually recommend a bone scan. Similarly, a bone scan is also recommended if a patient has a low PSA yet palpable disease and/or a Gleason score suggesting aggressive disease. A spot on a bone scan may be caused by cancer that has metastasized or by arthritis and other causes. When an abnormality shows up on a bone scan, further tests such as traditional X-rays, CT or MRI may be used to determine if the cause is cancer. It is important to establish a baseline to differentiate between cancer and other abnormalities.

Positron emission tomography (PET) is another technique that produces a 3-dimensional image of functional processes in the body. The system detects pairs of X-rays emitted indirectly by a positron-emitting tracer that is introduced into the body on a biologically active molecule. 3-dimensional images of tracer concentration in the body are then constructed by computer analysis. The 3-dimensional imaging is usually accomplished with the aid of a CT scan performed on the patient with the same machine.

Most of our patients undergo an Na F-18 PET/CT Fusion study, which has a predictive accuracy of 98% (Einat E et al., J Nucl Med 2006; 47:287-297). This avoids the false positive and false negative rates associated with bone scans (as a result of the F-18 tumor-imaging agent).

Again, bone scans and PET scans utilized in concert with other modalities enable us to more effectively treat prostate cancer, and thereby save lives.

What are the Risks of Immunodeficiency after Radiotherapy?

We are aware that a few doctors have recently issued irresponsible warnings about utilizing radiation therapy for lymph node disease associated with recurrent prostate cancer. They contend there is no evidence that radiation for lymph nodes has long-term survival benefits and they also warn that radiation therapy for these patients may carry a greater risk of developing bladder and colon cancer. But our own experience and that of other physicians who treat lymph node spread with radiation therapy strongly suggests that the opposite is true, that RT is both safe and effective for treating lymph nodes.

Radiation oncologists have been aware for many years that patients who are treated with radiation and subsequently undergo lymphocyte studies often show an apparent decline in immune system functions. One doctor outside the field of radiation oncology has even suggested that the post-radiation decline of CD3 and CD4 lymphocytes in prostate cancer patients is comparable to the decline seen with patients who develop AIDS. This reckless observation, circulated on the Internet and by word of mouth, has had a disastrous impact on some of our patients.

We have actually seen patients who locked themselves in to quarantine themselves in their apartments under the false impression that they might contract AIDS. We had one patient who was in treatment and because of his low CD3 and CD4 count, he locked himself in his condo and would only leave to come to our center for treatment. He was having food delivered because he didn't want to go outside and risk catching AIDS.

The reality is, as most of us in the field know, that with radiation therapy the CD3 and CD4 counts typically decline. But what happens with other cells in the immune system like the natural killer T-cells? These cells are far more powerful in terms of scouting around and taking care of the immune system than are the CD3 and CD4 lymphocytes. There is a decline in immune function of certain cells with patients having radiation, but it is counterbalanced by these memory T-cells that act like custodians of the immune system. This phenomenon is so profound that it engenders what may result in what is called an "abscopal effect." This means that when we treat one area of the body with radiation, it triggers a cascade of events that not only kills cancer in that specific area but travels to other parts of the body where cancer may have found sanctuary and eradicates it. These are areas of the body that are not even directly treated with radiation.

As a discipline, we know that patients do have declines in lymphocyte counts and if we check those counts constantly, they are going to be low but they will recover. In the right hands, there is certainly nothing dangerous about lymph node radiation in therapeutic doses. Lymph node radiation has been done for a long time. Up until recently, Hodgkin's Lymphoma patients had a single lymph node treated down to the groin. These patients have been tracked and followed extensively with studies from the Stanford Medical Center and the Memorial Sloan-Kettering Cancer Center, and they did not develop immunodeficiency diseases like AIDS.

There are studies that show these patients may have had a genetic predisposition to developing other cancers simply by virtue of having had Hodgkin's Lymphoma. Patients are also having their pelvic and rectal lymph nodes treated at a very young age. There is no data demonstrating that these patients develop diseases such as AIDS.

When women have breast cancer, we treat all of their lymph nodes with radiation going down and up into the neck, and they don't develop AIDS. After many decades of treating patients with radiation, we would certainly know by now if patients were contracting opportunistic infections due to radiation exposure. General practitioners would be noticing their patients coming down with serious diseases and looking at their histories to determine if at some point that they all had radiation as a common denominator. But that has never happened. So that is a myth circulated by a few irresponsible doctors, an untruth that is simply not supported by any studies.

With respect to the alleged damaging effects of radiation whereby the immune system becomes depleted and patients are said to be subject to infections of all kinds as with AIDS, one of the leading experts on immunology said in a private exchange with us, "The temporary reduction of T-cells resulting from radiation therapy is a very well known phenomenon to most radiation oncologists and medical oncologists. We are also aware of the abscopal effect, the indirect unexpected effects of radiation, which actually result in an anti-tumor immune response that appears to activate other systemic elements of the immune system. Researchers have identified tumor-related levels and antibody populations which support the fact that radiation triggers the system to fight locally but also at distant sights outside of the radiation field. Again, this is a temporary and well known phenomenon which apparently negates the decline to T-cell counts."

This physician went on to say that he was deeply concerned upon learning that some patients were being encouraged to essentially quarantine themselves following radiation of lymph nodes. These doctors who are crying wolf are also citing data erroneously to try to suggest there is no survival benefit to treating lymph nodes.

There was a study called RTOG 7506 for which researchers radiated retropubic and pelvic lymph nodes, and they found that they had an astounding ten-year survival with these patients, who would have been dead without treatment. Doctors in the past would say that if you had lymph node disease you should go home and put your affairs in order. But a sizeable number of those patients were alive at ten and fifteen years. Researchers at Memorial Sloan-Kettering Cancer Center published a study and that found that at fifteen years there was a 34% to 37% likelihood of patients surviving. That may sound like a low number, but these were patients who were deemed incurable. They were told that hormones were the only option that they had until they became resistant hormonal therapy and it stopped working.

There are a number of other statistically powerful studies from the standpoint of disease progression and cancer-free survival. They suggest that the cancers are not progressing after treatment of lymph node disease with radiation and the results translate into an overall survival, unlike what some of these doctors outside the field have suggested. There is another study called the Milan Match Analysis Trial, where surgery patients were treated with radiation combined with hormonal therapy and that study was statistically significant in terms of survival after ten years – 86% patient survival verses 70%. Statisticians understand that result is statistically very compelling, with less than 0.004 P value for survival (Briganti et al, European Urol, 59: 832-40, 2011).

Another study, RTOG 9202, also found that patients with Gleason 8-10 who had had lymph node disease would benefit significantly over time from an overall survival perspective after radiation therapy. These evidence-based studies show that there is indeed a survival benefit associated with treating lymph nodes. There was a famous European study led by Dr. Michel Bolla—the EORTC trial which was first published in 2009. He treated patients with advance disease; they were T-3 stage disease and higher and they received hormones and radiation. The results were quite impressive in terms of survival. We believe if they had tested the patients with advanced imaging, they would have found numerous involved lymph nodes.

What are the Risks of Secondary Cancers after Radiotherapy?

The risk of secondary bladder and rectal cancer many years after radiation treatment for prostate cancer is another controversial issue that has not yet been fully resolved. If a patient has prostate cancer, it involves the genital and urinary system and any patient who has prostate cancer is at risk for possibly developing renal cell cancer, which is cancer of the kidneys. Prostate cancer patients may also have a very small increased risk of developing bladder cancer, and increased risk of developing testicular cancer—these cancers are all part of the same system. This is not unique to prostate cancer. If we look at gynecological cancers, we seem the same thing: there is risk for cervical cancer and uterine cancer, because these cancers are part of GYN system for women, while in men, it's the GU system that carries a higher risk for cancers.

In July 2012, two studies were published by researchers at the Memorial Sloan-Kettering Cancer Center showing that with brachytherapy and Intensity Modulated Radiotherapy (IMRT) there was no increased risk for secondary bladder and colorectal cancers with patients who were followed 5 and 10 years. The incidence of secondary cancers for these patients treated with the most sophisticated forms of radiation therapy was no greater than that of the population at large and no greater than that of patients who had undergone radical surgery. One study also reported that the majority of the small number of patients who developed secondary malignancies were still alive 5 and 10 years after treatment (Zelefsky et al, BJU Int. 2012 Dec;110(11):1696-701. doi: 10.1111/j.1464-410X.2012.11385.x. Epub 2012 Aug 13 and Zelefsky et al, Int J Radiat Oncol Biol Phys. 2012 Jul 1;83(3):953-9.

A Canadian study in March 2016 analyzed 21 previous studies on the subject and reported a very small increased risk of secondary cancers with patients who had been treated with radiation. But even the researchers admitted that this study was flawed as were a number of the studies on which it was based, in part because the radiation delivery systems in the studies were essentially antiquated predating IMRT. In addition the authors failed to take into account other risk factors, such as smoking and alcohol consumption, by the patients who were followed in the various studies that were analyzed.

There are other papers that show in a very compelling way with colorectal cancers that as we follow the patients many years after treatment, they are getting older, and colorectal cancer is a very common cancer for that age group. So these patients may develop cancer at an increased rate as they get older, but most likely not because of radiation. If there is any risk at all, it is certainly very small.

We advise our patients to weigh that very minimal risk of secondary cancers against the benefits of radiation therapy, in order to decide on treating and eradicating their prostate cancer or allowing the disease to progress and become life threatening.

What Are The Results of The Dattoli Combined Protocol?

The treatment protocol combining brachytherapy with DART has been perfected by Dr. Dattoli and his team over a greater than 20-year period, and has produced **the longest and best published cure rate** in all the medical literature. With our current combination protocol, patients having low risk disease enjoy a greater than 95% biochemical success rate while, thanks to our advanced DART technology, we are now seeing even those patients having intermediate to high-risk disease achieving an approximate 90% cure rate with remarkably few, temporary side effects. Having treated patients with lymph node cancer and even bone metastases successfully, we are moving up the ladder in terms of the stage of the disease that can be conquered.

Our results have improved each year with refinements in technique and technology. As of 2010, our published data (*Journal of Oncology*, August, 2010) on patients with higher risk disease reported an 82% biochemical success rate with a follow up of 16 years. It is important to note that those patients were treated between 1992 and 1997 with combination of Palladium-103 brachytherapy and 3D Conformal Radiation Therapy, which during that decade was the most sophisticated form of external radiation therapy available. We have come a long way since that time with our current state-of-the-art DART capabilities and constantly improving seed implantation methods, translating into even more successful results.

The data that we published for higher risk patients is especially important because the vast majority of those patients treated in our 16-year series were considered incurable using any other treatment method, especially radical prostatectomy. To date, no other practitioners in the world have reported results as successful as our series with higher risk patients. As mentioned, the biochemical cure rate for low risk patients in our practice is typically greater than 95%, which is comparable or superior to the results achieved by the other leading brachytherapy teams. When treating intermediate and high risk disease, we simply have no equals.

Yet as impressive as the published results are, they do not reflect the effectiveness of our current technologies and skills. We believe our cure rates to be much higher, given the much higher doses that can be delivered with DART and the far greater accuracy, **which now enables us to most effectively eradicate the cancer while minimizing side effects—and we accomplish this one patient at a time.**

Summary of the Dattoli 16-year Data

The following summary is based on a Dattoli series that was first presented at an American Society of Clinical Oncology meeting (February, 2009), and sub-sequently published in the *Journal of Oncology* (Dattoli M, Wallner K True L, Bostwick D, Cash J, Sorace, R, Long-term Outcomes for Patients with Prostate Cancer having Intermediate and High-risk Disease, treated with Brachytherapy and Supplemental External Beam Radiotherapy, J Oncol. 2010; pii: 471375. Epub 2010 Aug 18). The summary also draws on an earlier published series (Dattoli M, et al., *Urology*, 2007 Feb; 69(2):334-337).

The bottom line in our studies is that these are patients who were at high risk, with a high likelihood of extra-capsular extension (cancer that has spread outside the prostate gland). These patients were treated with 3D-Conformal Radiation (which was the state-of-the-art approach prior to the IMRT era) followed by seed implantation, with large margins. The study was by a single author-practitioner doing the implants, but the biochemical data was independently reviewed by the University of Washington, and all the slides were re-reviewed by the University of Washington, which adds an element of security to the data. Clinical stage was not included because the doctors at the University of Washington couldn't perform a digital rectal exam on these patients due to geographical distance. It should be noted that we have been following many patients from this series and others for more than 20 years. We have not seen any evidence to suggest that our combined treatment protocol has led to secondary malignancies or infections caused by immunodeficiency.

For the most part in our practice, side effects following DART with or without brachytherapy are only temporary and manageable, as reported in our published studies.

The 16-year Data—*Summary*

Materials and Methods
321 Consecutive Patients treated by one author (M.D.)—157 intermediate risk and 164 high risk.

Selection Criteria
NCCN Guidelines

Radiation Treatment Regimen
- 3D-CRT Dose: 4140cGy Median (Range 39 Gy–54 Gy)
- Pd-103 Dose: 8000-9000 Minimum Peripheral Dose (pre-NIST-99)
- Source Strength: 1.4 mCi Median (Range 1.1-1.6 mCi)
- Clinical Pd-103 Target Volume: extended 0.5 – 1.0 cm, antero-laterally to the TRUS prostate margin
- Patients were followed at 3, 6 and 12 months, and every 6-12 months thereafter
- Definition of biochemical success: PSA $\leq$ 0.2 ng/ml, nadir +2 and ASTRO Consensus Definition
- Follow-up saturation prostate biopsies were performed on all failing patients
- Biochemical data independently re-reviewed and analyzed by Kent Wallner, MD (Univ. of Washington)
- Original biopsy slides re-reviewed by Lawrence True, MD (Univ. of Washington)
- Clinical stage was not included in final data analysis to reduce subjectivity

Patient Characteristics
- Mean PSA 19.4 (1.6–147)
- Median PSA 16.4
- 218 Patients had Gleason Score 7-10
- 203 Patients had PSA > 10
- 79 Patients had elevated PAPs
- 141 Patients had Clinical Stage T2C
- 127 Patients had Clinical Stage T3

Follow-up
- 16 year actuarial, Median 10.3 years
- 143 Patients received a median of 4 months neo-adjuvant or adjuvant therapy

Results
- PAP was the strongest predictor of failure (p= 0.0001), followed by Gleason Score (p< 0.001) and PSA (p=0.03)
- Hormones conferred no survival advantage (p=0.4) although patients receiving hormones had the most adverse features
- 82% overall actuarial freedom from biochemical progress at 16 years using strict PSA nadir of ≤0.2 ng/ml (Freedom from failure calculated by method of Kaplan-Meier. Difference between groups were determined by the log rank or students' t-test) (86% cancer specific survival; 89% intermediate and 74% high risk)
- The absolute risk of failure fell to 1% beyond 5 years after treatment
- Treatment morbidity was limited to RTOG grade 1-2 symptoms. No patients experienced grade 3-4 toxicity. (One patient who had both a TURP and TUIP developed low-volume stress incontinence.) No patient developed rectal ulceration
- All failing patients underwent prostatic biopsies. There were no pathologically documented local failures

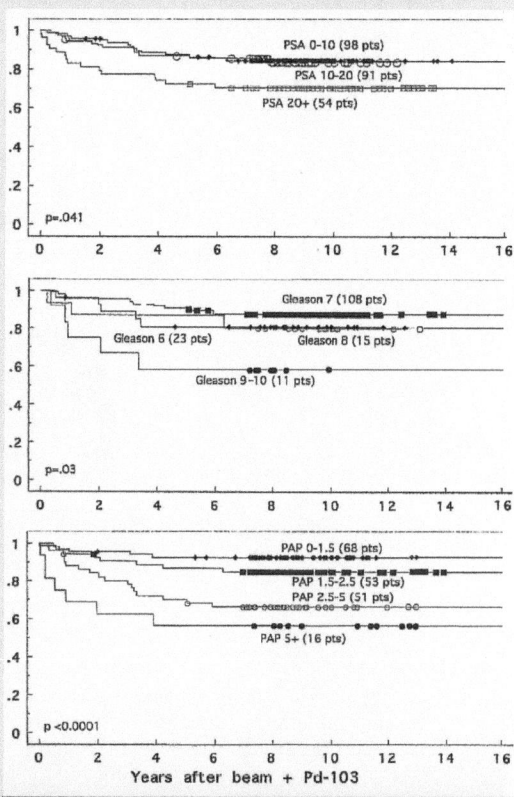

These three graphs show the freedom of biographical progression of the disease out to 16 years stratified by PSA, Gleason Score, and PAP.

Conclusions

- Patients having high risk prostate cancer may enjoy long-term biochemical freedom even when using strict PSA nadirs
- Morbidity has been very acceptable
- Despite the aggressive nature of this study group, no local failures have been documented
- It is encouraging that the failure rate decreased to near zero with follow-up beyond 5 years
- These results appear superior to surgery, aggressive external beam radiotherapy (including full course IMRT ± hormones, protons/neutrons or combined radiation methods using other isotopes ± hormones) in this high risk group
- We attribute these exceedingly favorable results, in part, to our effort to achieve wide brachytherapy treatment margins. This is accomplished by using highly peripheral and extra-capsular source placement
- PD-103 appears to be the isotope best suited for high-risk cancers

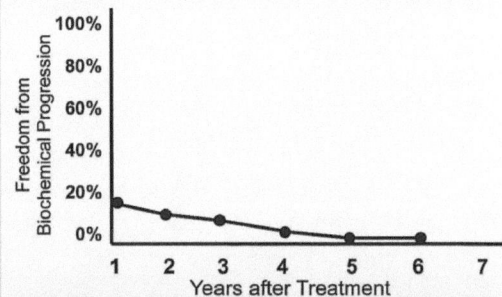

This graph shows the likelihood of subsequent bio-chemical failure versus years after treatment. These results are encouraging because as time goes on fewer and fewer patients experience biochemical failure, indicated by a PSA greater than 0.2.

APPENDIX A

PUBLISHED COMMENTARY ON EVALUATING RADIATION SAFETY

Replacing LNT: The Integrated LNT-Hormesis Model

Kaminski CY, Dattoli MJ, and Kaminski, JM,
Dose Response. 2020 Apr 15;18(2):1559325820913788.

Abstract

Many scientists and regulators utilize the linear no-threshold (LNT) relationship to estimate the likelihood of carcinogenesis. The LNT model is incorrect and was adopted based upon false pretenses. The use of the model has been corrupted by many to claim that even the smallest ionizing radiation dose may initiate carcinogenesis. This claim has resulted in societal harm.

Introduction

The linear no-threshold (LNT) model is based upon the proportionality of radiation dose and cancer risk. This model is supported by flawed scientific and epidemiological data. For example, the scientific data, based upon γH2AX foci as a marker for DNA double-strand breakage, demonstrate linearity between dose and DNA damage from 1 mGy to 100 Gy. The hypotheses follow: (1) Each double-strand break has an equal probability at inducing transformation irrespective of the number of double-strand breaks simultaneously within the cell and (2) each transformed cell has the same probability of developing into a cancer irrespective of the tissue environment and/or health of the organism.[1, 2] However, γH2AX is a nonspecific marker and may result from single-strand breaks.[3]

From the scientific data, one must conclude that dose and carcinogenic risk is nonlinear if one views the organism in a hierarchical approach. Organisms are made up of systems, systems are made up of tissues, tissues are made up of cells, and cells are made up of their constituents. At each level mechanisms exist to prevent and/or mitigate damage. [4-6]

Cellular Defenses

Three types of defenses that immediately combat DNA damage have been identified.[7] (1) Defenses against reactive oxygen species (ROS)—Oxygen metabolism, infection, physical exercise, ionizing radiation, ultraviolet light, chemicals, and others result in ROS. Potential damage is mitigated by scavengers and antioxidant molecules within cells. (2) DNA repair—There are cellular sensor molecules that detect DNA damage which eventually result in cell cycle arrest, DNA repair, and upregulation of defense mechanisms. DNA repair is dependent upon the dose and dose rate. (3) Elimination of damaged cells—Cells are eliminated through apoptotic, mitotic, and senescent cell death.

Adaptive Responses

When cells undergo radiogenic or nonradiogenic genotoxic damage, an increase in protective mechanisms are observed in the cells and nearby cells (bystander effects). These defenses include ROS scavengers, damaged cell removal, and DNA repair. The upregulation of these factors can last for hours to months. [7]

Tissue Defenses

The surrounding environment protects and controls cellular proliferation when functional. If the microenvironment is impaired through physical, chemical agents, or disease, the cells are more likely to undergo DNA alterations with subsequent neoplastic transformation. Tissue disorganization also facilitates escape of preneoplastic subclones from microenvironmental barriers. For example, fibrosis increases the risk for cancer of the lung, liver, and skin. Immune mechanisms are also potent regulators in the prevention of cancer. Currently, there are many therapies that modulate the immune system for the treatment of cancer.

Although an imperfect system, life has evolved to protect itself from genotoxic damage. When cellular and/or tissue repair mechanisms are damaged, the risk of cancer increases. Organisms are constantly undergoing genotoxic stresses. Small insults are fairly well addressed and may be beneficial; however, with large insults, the cell, the tissue, the system, and the body are unable to compensate appropriately and the risk of cancer exceeds a threshold above which cancer risk increases.

Too often, epidemiological evidence is used inappropriately to support the LNT model. For example, the atomic bomb data have been frequently used to demonstrate the concept of the LNT model. However, the atomic bomb survivors were exposed to other carcinogenic agents including trauma from nonradioactive insults such as burns, nonradioactive toxins from the explosion, and subsequent fires, which contaminated the food, water, and air.[8] Environmental stressors unrelated to ionizing radiation increase the risk for carcinogenesis or other adverse health effects. For example, the World Trade Center Disaster on September 11, 2001, released a number of toxins into the environment possibly resulting in an increased risk of certain cancers.[9]

Also, the incidence of all cancers was higher among Israeli Jews who were exposed to the extreme stressors of the Holocaust than among those who were not.[10] These nonradioactive stressors should be considered by those claiming that low doses of radiation are carcinogenic. Furthermore, the stigma associated with the radioactive exposure may have resulted in many atomic bomb survivors who were exposed to higher doses to claim that they were further away from the explosion, resulting in incorrect dose estimates. To further complicate the matter, the estimated doses do not include that from residual radiation thereby underestimating those (including the "not in the city" control population) who were thought to have received, for example, less than 100 mGy.[11-12] Furthermore, the atomic bomb survivors and the "not in the city" controls have a longer life span and reduced cancer mortality relative to unirradiated Japanese.[12] There are many good reviews that provide critiques of the epidemiological studies.[7, 13, 14]

Hormesis

Compelling scientific and epidemiological data for hormesis exist.[13-19] Small insults, whether from radiation or other genotoxic stressors, result in upregulation of protective mechanism at the cell and tissue level. These defenses more than compensate for any potential (or real) damage that the organism incurred from the original insult; thereby decreasing the risk of carcinogenesis from future genotoxic insults.

Conclusion

Data for ionizing radiation induced carcinogenesis support the existence of a hormetic response at low doses with a threshold. The dose from current diagnostic studies (e.g., 10 mGy) is well below the threshold. Those who estimate radiation induced cancer risks should consider confounding effects of coexisting nonradiation carcinogenic risks. The fear of carcinogenesis that has been propagated due to those grossly overestimating the cancer risks from low doses of ionizing radiation is unethical and has resulted in medical, economic, and other societal harm.[20-24] harm.The LNT model should not be applied for cancer risks in the low-dose range. The regulatory bodies including the Nuclear Regulatory Commission should change from an LNT model based risk assessment to the integrated LNT-Hormesis model as Calabrese describes.[25]

References

1. NCRP. Evaluation of the Linear-Nonthreshold Dose-Response Model for Ionizing Radiation. Bethesda, MD: NCRP, 2001: NCRP Report No. 136.
2. NCRP. Implications of Recent Epidemiological Studies for the Linear-Nonthreshold Model and Radiation Protection. Bethesda, MD: NCRP, 2018: NCRP Commentary No. 27.
3. Katsube T, Mori M, Tsuji H. Most hydrogen peroxide-induced histone H2AX phosphorylation is mediated by ATR and is not dependent on DNA double-strand breaks. J Biochem. 2014; 156(2):85-95.
4. Feinendegen LE, Pollycove M, Neumann RD. Whole-body responses to low-level radiation exposure: new concepts in mammalian radiobiology. Exp Hematol. 2007;35(4 suppl 1):37-46.
5. Trosko JE. Hierarchical and cybernetic nature of biologic systems and their relevance to homeostatic adaptation to low-level exposures to oxidative stress-inducing agents. Environ Health Perspect. 1998;106(suppl 1):331-339.
6. Ulsh BA. Checking the foundation: recent radiobiology and the linear no-threshold theory. Health Phys. 2010;99(6):747-758.
7. Tubiana M, Feinendegen LE, Yang C, Kaminski JM. The linear no-threshold relationship is inconsistent with radiation biologic and experimental data. Radiology. 2009;251(1):13-22.
8. Institute of Medicine (US) Steering Committee for the Symposium on the Medical Implications of Nuclear War. Solomon F, Marston RQ, eds. The Medical Implications of Nuclear War. Washington, DC: National Academies Press (US); 1986. Possible Toxic Environments Following a Nuclear War. https://www.ncbi.nlm.nih.gov/books/NBK219160/. Accessed March 16, 2020.
9. Lieberman-Cribbin W, Tuminello S, Gillezeau C, et al. The development of a Biobank of cancer tissue samples from World Trade Center responders. J Transl Med. 2018;16(1):280.
10. Keinan-Boker L, Vin-Raviv N, Liphshitz I, Linn S, Barchana M. Cancer incidence in Israeli Jewish survivors of World War II. J Natl Cancer Inst. 2009;101(21):1489-1500.
11. Sutou S. Rediscovery of an old article reporting that the area around the epicenter in Hiroshima was heavily contaminated with residual radiation, indicating that exposure doses of A-bomb survivors were largely underestimated. J Radiat Res. 2017;58(5): 745-754.
12. Sutou S. Low-dose radiation from A-bombs elongated lifespan and reduced cancer mortality relative to un-irradiated individuals [published correction appears in Genes Environ. 2019 Apr 19;41:12]. Genes Environ. 2018;40:26. doi:10.1186/s41021-018-0114-3.
13. Scott BR. A critique of recent epidemiologic studies of cancer mortality among nuclear workers. Dose Response. 2018;16(2): 1559325818778702.
14. Shibamoto Y, Nakamura H. Overview of biological, epidemiological, and clinical evidence of radiation hormesis. Int J Mol Sci. 2018;19(8):2387. doi:10.3390/ijms19082387.
15. Calabrese EJ. Hormesis: path and progression to significance. Int J Mol Sci. 2018;19(10):2871.
16. Cardarelli JJ II, Ulsh BA. It is time to move beyond the linear no-threshold theory for low-dose radiation protection. Dose Response. 2018;16(3):1559325818779651.
17. Cuttler JM, Feinendegen LE. Commentary on inhaled (239)PUO2 in Dogs—a prophylaxis against lung cancer? Dose Response. 2015;13(1).pii: dose–response.15–003.Cuttler.
18. Cuttler JM, Sanders CL. Threshold for radon-induced lung cancer from inhaled plutonium data. Dose Response. 2015;13(4): 1559325815615102.
19. Pennington CW, Siegel JA. The Linear no-threshold model of low-dose radiogenic cancer: a failed fiction. Dose Response. 2019; 17(1):1559325818824200.
20. Akabayashi A, Hayashi Y. Mandatory evacuation of residents during the Fukushima nuclear disaster: an ethical analysis. J Public Health (Oxf). 2012;34(3):348-351.
21. Hasegawa A, Tanigawa K, Ohtsuru A. Health effects of radiation and other health problems in the aftermath of nuclear accidents, with an emphasis on Fukushima. Lancet. 2015;386(9992): 479-488.
22. Murakami M, Ono K, Tsubokura M. Was the risk from nursinghome evacuation after the Fukushima accident higher than the radiation risk? PLoS One. 2015;10(9):e0137906.
23. Wigg DR. Radiation: facts, fallacies and phobias. Australas Radiol. 2007;51(1):21-25.
24. Yasumura S, Goto A, Yamazaki S, Reich MR. Excess mortality among relocated institutionalized elderly after the Fukushima nuclear disaster. Public Health. 2013;127(2):186-188.
25. Calabrese EJ. Model uncertainty via the integration of hormesis and LNT as the default in cancer risk assessment. Dose Response. 2015;13(4):1559325815621764.

APPENDIX B

DECIDING WHAT IS BEST FOR YOU

Consult with your physician, and by all means, obtain second and third opinions whenever possible, preferably from physicians with different specialties. If you have already been to a urologist, it is worthwhile to visit a radiation oncologist or medical oncologist (those with experience with hormones and chemotherapy).

Join a support group such as US TOO!, or PAACT. If you belong to any of the computer on-line services, check out the medical and health bulletin boards and mailing lists for the latest information and announcements for prostate cancer patients. Keep your personal plan of action updated.

What to Remember

- Obtain all of the advice and counsel that you can, but keep in mind that the decisions are ultimately yours to make.

- Be positive—if you have been properly staged and treated, the odds are in your favor on not having a recurrence.

- If you should have a rising PSA over time after initial treatment, don't panic. Get further tests, and if appropriate, get a biopsy, preferably guided by color flow Doppler ultrasound.

- The secret to success with prostate cancer is catching the disease early, and that is also true for recurrence.

- If testing confirms cancer, learn all you can about your options. Get second and third opinions. Become informed and empowered. Become involved with solving your problem. It's your life and body. Go for it!

- Life is full of problems and challenges. Solve this problem like any other big problem:
    1. Identify the problem.
    2. Get all the facts to confirm that you have a problem.
    3. Learn what options are available to you and weigh them carefully.
    4. Choose a qualified doctor who is experienced and with whom you are comfortable.
    5. Initiate and follow through with the solution.
- Don't be afraid to ask for help from your spouse or partner, from your family and your friends. It is more important than ever for you to turn to loved ones to get the emotional and spiritual support you need. This disease can be a difficult struggle for us, but we are not alone, and our mental attitude, prayers and our fighting spirit really can make all the difference.

To be a cancer survivor, you must first be a cancer fighter!

APPENDIX C

ADVANCED IMAGING AND TREATMENT PLANNING AT THE DATTOLI CANCER CENTER AND BRACHYTHERAPY INSTITUTE

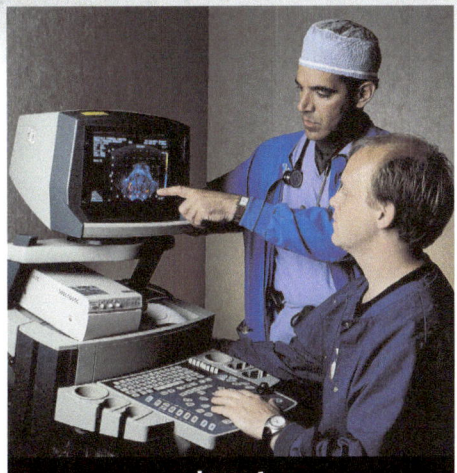

Image 1
3-Dimensional color-flow Doppler ultrasound is used to image cancer areas inside and outside the prostate gland. At our center, patients are invited to view their color-flow Doppler ultrasound images in order to visualize the treatment process.

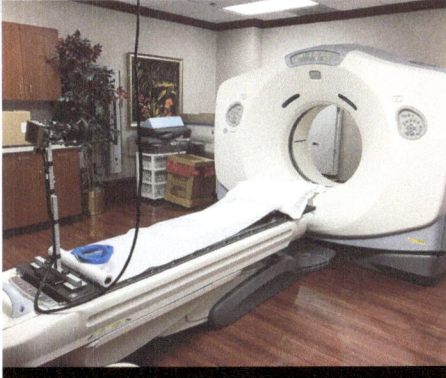

Image 2
The GE High Speed Helical CT Scanner captures high resolution images of the prostate, seminal vesicles, bladder, urethra and rectum, required to accurately design an individual treatment plan. The GE Scanner is also equipped to perform baseline and follow-up QCT Bone Density evaluations.

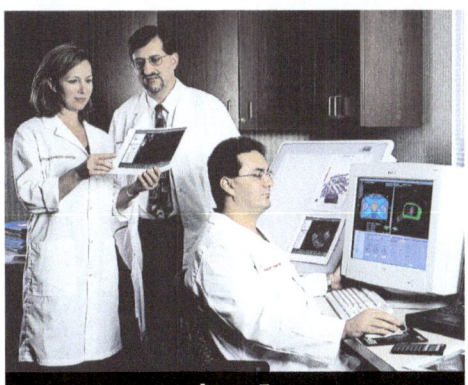

Image 3
The computer center for planning and customizing the best treatment programs utilizing brachytherapy and Image-Guided Intensity Modulated Radiation Therapy (IG-IMRT)

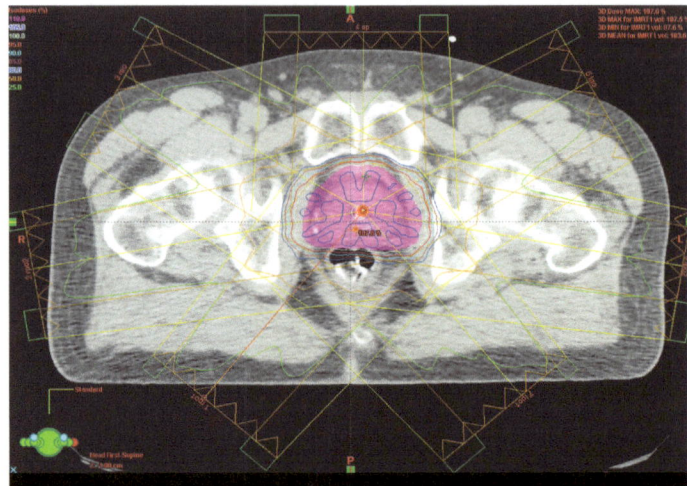

Image 11
We tell the computer what dose we want to direct to the volume of interest and what dose limits we want for the surrounding structures such as the bladder and rectum. The computer gives us the best possible plan which in this view is displayed as isodose lines around the volume of interest. Each line represents a percentage of the dose as outlined in the key in the upper left corner.

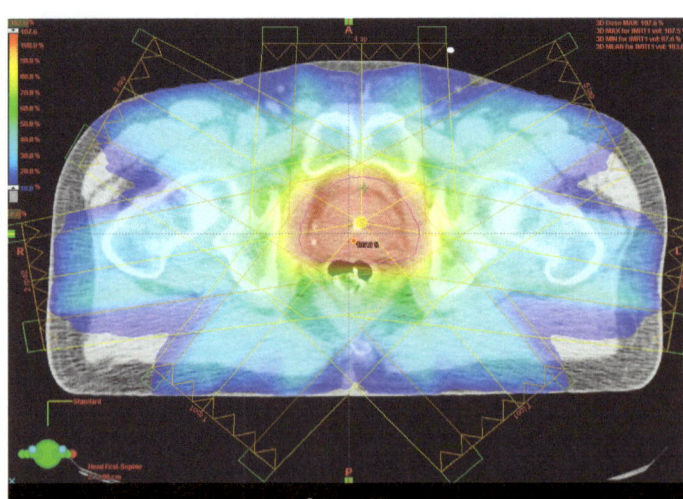

Image 12
This is the same as the previous image but shown in a color wash mode. You can see that where all of the 7 fields converge is where the dose is the "hottest" (color red) and where the dose is "cooler" (color blue). This shows nice uniform coverage around the volume of interest (purple line).

APPENDIX C: ADVANCED IMAGING AND TREATMENT PLANNING AT DATTOLI CANCER CENTER

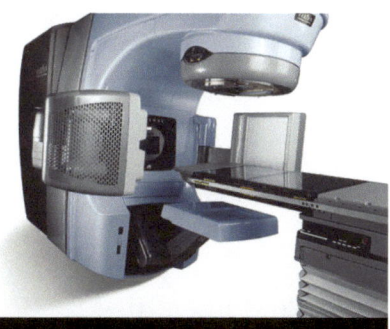

Image 13
A linear accelerator for delivering 4D IG-IMRT with DART, complete with on-board imaging capabilities and the 'exact couch' system.

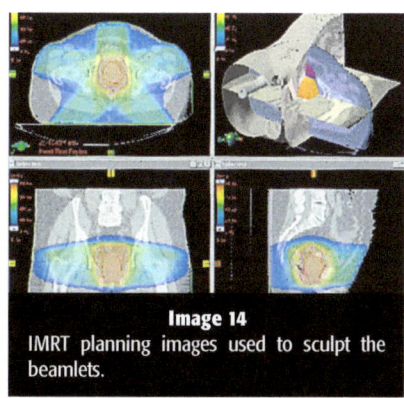

Image 14
IMRT planning images used to sculpt the beamlets.

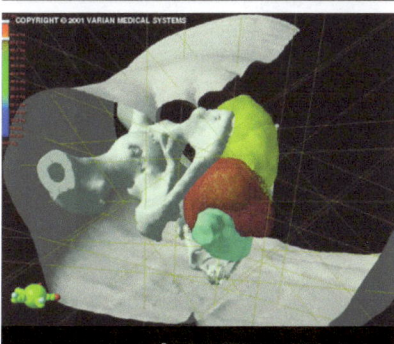

Image 15
An IMRT plan for treating prostate cancer, concentrating the radiation dose in the tumor (red) while avoiding the nearby bladder (yellow) and rectum (green). Courtesy of Varian Medical Systems.

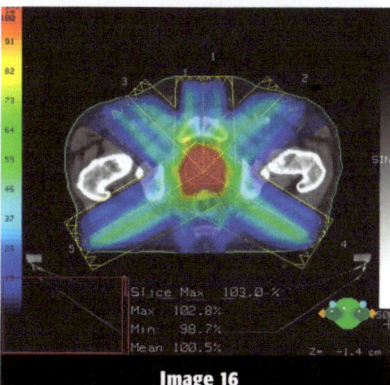

Image 16
A color-wash representation of an IMRT plan, showing how the radiation dose will be distributed in and around the prostate. The area of high dose (red) corresponds tightly to the tumor area being treated. Courtesy of Varian Medical Systems.

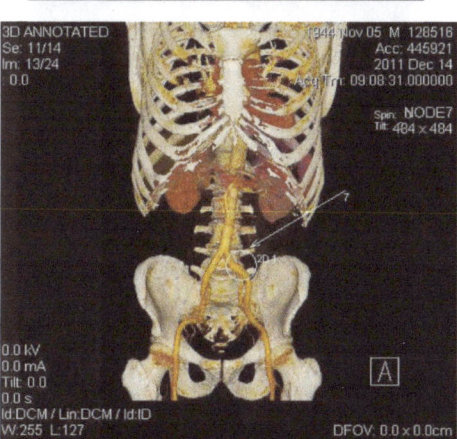
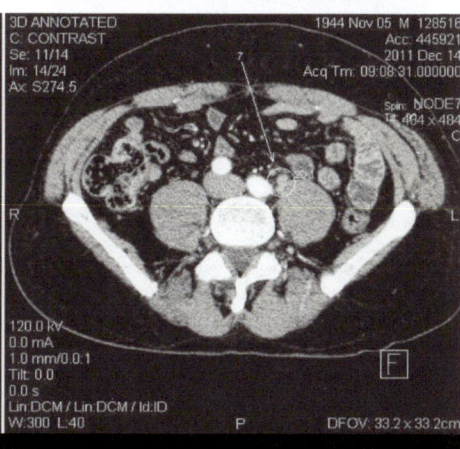

Image 17
A Dynamic Contrast Enhanced MRI study for the identification of cancer metastasis in the lymph nodes.

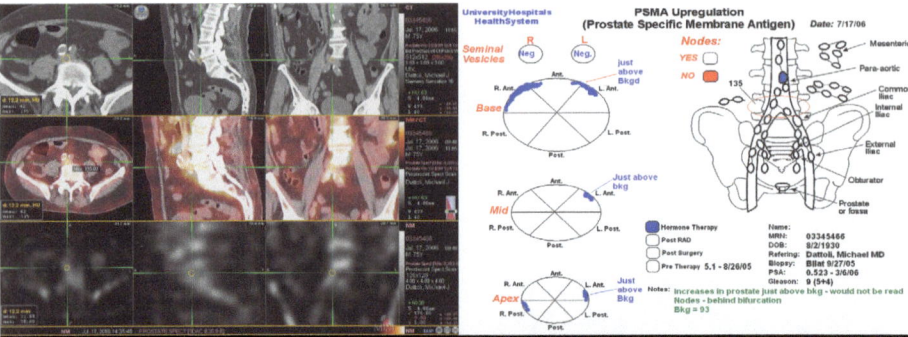

Images 18
ProstaScint® is another diagnostic test that enables doctors to determine lymph node involvement. ProstaScint® can be fused with helical CT or with MRI or with CT/PET scans. A pictorial analysis for this patient appears to the right of the scanned images.

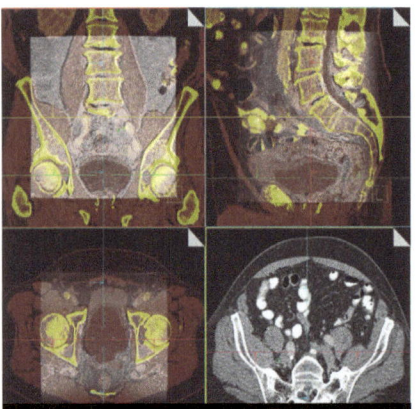

Image 19
The first three images (top right/left and bottom left) are of the abdomen and pelvis in saggital, coronal and axial views. They are MRI fused images that highlight bony anatomy and enhance organs with a rich blood supply. On the first of these images, you can see the right and left kidneys in the upper part of the frame. The last of the four images (bottom right) is a CT scan of the abdomen used to correlate with the fused MRI images for reference.

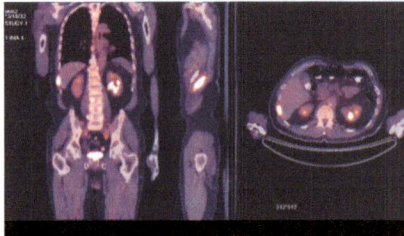

Image 20
The 18F-Fluoride PET/CT imaging technique has demonstrated 100% predictive accuracy (sensitivity and specificity), which is as good as it gets. The images show a biopsy-proven skeletal lesion (metastatic prostate cancer) in one rib, which proved to be treatable. We've pushed the envelope with respect to where we can treat, because the technologies are now so advanced.

APPENDIX D

GLOSSARY OF MEDICAL TERMS

3D-CRT (3-Dimensional Conformal Radiation Therapy): See Conformal Radiotherapy.

5-alpha reductase (5-AR): an enzyme that converts testosterone to dihydrotestosterone (DHT).

Adenocarcinoma: A cancer originating in glandular tissue. Prostate cancer is classified as adenocarcinoma of the prostate.

Adjuvant: An additional treatment used to increase the effectiveness of the primary therapy. Radiation therapy and hormonal therapy are often used as adjuvant treatments following a radical prostatectomy. Compare Neoadjuvant.

Agonist: A chemical substance that combines with a receptor on a cell and initiates an activity or reaction. See LHRH analogs.

Algorithm: A step-by-step procedure for solving a problem or accomplishing some end, especially by a computer.

Analog: A man-made chemical compound that is structurally similar to one produced naturally by the body. See LHRH analogs.

Anastomotic stricture: narrowing, usually by scarring, of an anastomotic suture line.

Androgen: A hormone that produces male characteristics. See testosterone.

Androgen ablation therapy: A therapy designed to inhibit the body's production of testosterones.

Androgen-dependent cells: Prostate cancer cells which are nourished by male hormones and therefore are capable of being destroyed by hormone deprivation (also known as androgen-sensitive cells).

Androgen-independent cells: Prostate cancer cells which are not dependent on male hormones and therefore do not respond to hormonal therapy (also known as androgen-insensitive cells).

Anesthetic: A drug that produces general or local loss of physical sensations, particularly pain. A "spinal" is the injection of a local anesthetic into the area surrounding the spinal cord.

Aneuploid: Having an abnormal number of chromosomes, as revealed by ploidy analysis. Aneuploid prostate cancer cells tend not to respond well to androgen deprivation therapy (ADT).

Angiogenesis: The body's formation of new blood vessels. Some anti-cancer drugs work by blocking angiogenesis, thus preventing blood from reaching and nourishing a tumor.

Antagonist: A chemical substance in the body that acts to reduce the physiological activity of another chemical substance.

Antiandrogens: Drugs such as Casodex that block the activity of androgens produced by the adrenal glands at the cellular receptor sites. Androgens can block or neutralize the effects of testosterone and DHT on prostate cancer cells.

Antibody: A protein produced by the body that counteracts the toxic effects of a foreign substance, organism, or disease within the body.

Antigen: A foreign substance such as a virus or bacterium that causes an immune response or the formation of an antibody.

Antineoplastic: Inhibits growth and proliferation of cancer cells.

Antioxidants: Any substances which delay the process of oxidation in the body.

Apoptosis: The normal molecular mechanism which governs the life span of cells so that they die in a very organized way. Cancerous cells are resistant to normal apoptosis.

Benign: A non-cancerous condition. See also Benign Prostatic Hypertrophy.

Benign Prostatic Hypertrophy (BPH): Also called Benign Prostatic Hyperplasia, BPH is a non-cancerous condition of the prostate that results in a growth of tumorous tissue and increase in the size of the prostate.

Biopsy: A procedure involving the removal of tissue from the body of the patient. Removed tissue is typically examined microscopically by a pathologist in order to make a precise diagnosis of the patient's condition.

Bone scan: An imaging technique used to detect bone metastases, which appear as "hot spots" on the film. It is far more sensitive than the conventional x-ray.

BPH: See Benign Prostatic Hypertrophy.

Brachytherapy: A form of radiation therapy in which radioactive seeds are implanted into the prostate to deliver radiation directly to the tumor. Also referred to as seed implantation, or seeding.

Cancer: A cellular malignancy typically forming tumors. Unlike benign tumors, these tend to invade surrounding tissues and spread to distant sites of the body.

Carcinoma: A malignant tumor made up chiefly of epithelial cells, or those cells that form the lining of an organ or cavity. See Adenocarcinoma.

Castrate Range: The level of the body's testosterone after orchiectomy (also referred to as castration). This is the range or level, which is used by physicians as a point of comparison for those drugs, which attempt to decrease the testosterone level.

CAT Scan (or CT Scan): See Computer Tomography.

cGy: Abbreviation for centigray; a unit of radiation equivalent to the older unit called a "rad."

Chemotherapy: The treatment of cancer using chemicals that deter the growth of cancer cells.

Collimator: A device that organizes radiation such that only parallel rays or beams emanate.

Combination Hormonal Therapy (CHT): Also referred to as Combined Hormonal Blockade (CHB), or Combined Androgen Deprivation Therapy (ADT). The preferred term is ADT, often designated with a number referring to the number of agents used (i.e., monotherapy ADT, ADT2, ADT3). This combined therapy can utilize a number of mechanisms, including surgical or medical ADT, antiandrogens, 5-alpha reductase inhibitors, estrogenic compounds, agents that block adrenal androgen production, and agents that decrease the receptivity of the androgen receptor.

Combination Therapy: Refers generally to any combination of treatment modalities used to treat prostate cancer.

Computer Tomography: Computer generated cross-sectional images of a portion of the body. Also called CT or CAT scan.

Conformal Radiotherapy: A radiation treatment conforming precisely to the size and shape of the prostate, with the use of computerized planning and state-of-the-art imaging techniques. 3-Dimensional Conformal Radiation Therapy (3D-CRT) utilizes this sophisticated approach to treatment planning, as does the even more advanced Intensity Modulated Radiation Therapy (IMRT).

Cryosurgery (also referred to as Cryotherapy or Cryoablation): The freezing of tissue with the use of liquid nitrogen or Argon gas probes. When used to treat prostate cancer, the cryoprobes are guided by transrectal ultrasound.

Cytokine: Any of a class of immunoregulatory substances that are secreted by cells of the immune system.

DHT (dihydrotestosterone): The active form of the male hormone, testosterone, produced after testosterone is transformed by an enzyme known as 5-alpha reductase.

Diagnosis: Evaluation of a patient's symptoms and/or test results, with the intent of identifying and verifying the existence of any underlying disease or abnormal condition.

Digital Rectal Examination (DRE): A procedure in which the physician inserts a gloved, lubricated finger into the rectum to examine the prostate gland for signs of cancer.

DNA (Deoxyribonucleic Acid): A complex protein that is the carrier of genetic information that determines the physical development and growth of living organisms.

Doppler Ultrasound Technique: A machine that sends out ultrasonic waves that pick up the velocity of blood flow through the veins and are transmitted as sound to make an image.

Doubling Time: The time it takes for a tumor or cancerous focus to double in size.

Downsizing: The use of hormonal therapy or other forms of intervention to reduce tumor volume prior to primary, curative treatment.

Downstaging: The use of hormonal therapy or other forms of intervention to lower the clinical stage of prostate cancer prior to primary, curative treatment.

Ejaculatory Ducts: The tubular passages through which semen reaches the prostatic urethra during orgasm.

Ejaculation: The release of semen through the penis during orgasm.

Endorectal MRI: Magnetic resonance imaging of the prostate gland using a probe inserted into the rectum. Dynamic Contrast Enhanced MRI is the most effective form of magnetic resonance imaging.

Enzyme: A chemical substance produced by living cells that causes chemical reactions to take place while not being changed itself.

Erectile Dysfunction (also referred to as ED or impotence): The loss of ability to produce and/or sustain an erection sufficient for intercourse.

Estrogen: A female sex hormone that can be used as a form of therapy to inhibit the production of testosterone in patients diagnosed with prostate. cancer.

APPENDIX D: GLOSSARY OF MEDICAL TERMS

External Beam Radiation Therapy (EBRT): A form of radiation therapy that utilizes radiation delivered by an external source (machine) and directed at a target area to be radiated. In contrast to EBRT, brachytherapy utilizes radiation sources (seeds) that are internal, implanted in the target tissue. EBRT may use conventional photons, protons, neutrons or electrons.

Extraprostatic Extension: Used to describe prostate cancer that has spread outside the prostate gland.

False Negative: An erroneous negative test result. For example, an imaging test that fails to show the presence of a cancer tumor later found by biopsy to be present in the patient is said to have returned a false negative result.

False Positive: A positive test result that mistakenly identifies a state or condition that does not in fact exist.

Feraheme (Ferumoxytol): A ferromagnetic nanoparticle which is taken up by normal macrophages with the lymph nodes.

Fistula: With regard to prostate cancer, an abnormal passage due to injury or disease that connects an abscess or hollow organ to the surface of the body or to another hollow organ. If there is significant damage to the rectal wall proximate to the bladder, a fistula may occur between the bladder and rectum.

Flare Reaction: A testosterone surge caused by the initial use of an LHRH analog, causing a temporary increase of tumor growth and symptoms (known as clinical flare), or an increase in PSA (biochemical flare).

Foley Catheter: A catheter inserted in the penis and threaded through the urethra to the bladder where it is held in place with a tiny, inflated balloon. It removes urine from the bladder and can be used to irrigate the urethra and prevent blood clots.

Free PSA: PSA that is unattached to any major protein in the blood. Free PSA is associated with benign prostate growth. The percentage of free PSA is derived by dividing the free-PSA level by the total-PSA x 100. Studies have show that men with free PSA % > 25% were at low risk for prostate cancer, while men with PSA % < 10% were at high risk for having prostate cancer.

Frozen Section: A technique in which removed tissue is frozen, cut into thin slices, and stained for microscopic examination. A pathologist can rapidly complete a frozen section analysis, and for this reason, it is commonly used during surgery to quickly provide the surgeon with vital information.

Gland: An aggregation of cells (a structure or organ) that secretes a substance for use or discharge from the body.

Gland Volume: The size in cubic centimeters (cc) or grams of the prostate gland.

Gleason Score: A widely used method for classifying the cellular differentiation of cancerous tissue. The less the cancerous cells appear like normal cells, the more malignant the cancer. Two grades of 1-5, identifying the two most common degrees of differentiation present in the examined tissue sample, are added together to produce the Gleason score. High numbers indicate greater differentiation and more aggressive cancer. The grading system is named after its originator, Donald Gleason, M.D.

Globulin: Any of a number of simple proteins that occur widely in plant and animal tissues.

Gynecomastia: A side effect involving breast enlargement and tenderness, associated with various hormonal therapies that increase the level of estrogens in the body.

HDR brachytherapy: High Dose Rate brachytherapy involves the temporary insertion of radioactive iridium isotopes into the prostate gland using transrectal ultrasound guidance.

Hematuria: Blood in the urine.

Hereditary: Inherited genetically from parents and earlier generations.

Holistic Medicine: Medical care, which considers the patient as a whole, including his or her physical, mental, emotional, spiritual, social and economic needs.

Hormone: A substance produced by one tissue or gland and transported by the bloodstream to another to effect or regulate physiological activity such as metabolism and growth.

Hormonal therapy: Cancer treatment involving the blockage of hormone production by surgical or chemical means. Because prostate cancer is usually dependent on male hormones to grow, hormonal therapy can be an effective means of alleviating symptoms and retarding the development of the disease.

Hormone refractory prostate cancer: Prostate cancer that is androgen independent, and therefore, unresponsive to hormonal therapies.

Hot Flash: A side effect of some forms of hormonal therapy, experienced as a sudden rush of warmth to the face, neck, and upper body.

Imaging: Radiology techniques that are often computer-enhanced and allow the physician to visualize areas inside the body that would not normally be visible.

Impotence: See Erectile Dysfunction.

Incontinence: A loss of urinary control. There are various kinds and degrees of incontinence. Overflow incontinence is a condition in which the bladder retains urine after voiding. As a consequence, the bladder remains full most of the time, resulting in involuntary seepage of urine from the bladder. Stress incontinence is the involuntary discharge of urine when there is increased pressure upon the bladder, as in coughing or straining to lift heavy objects. Total incontinence is the failure of ability to voluntarily exercise control over the sphincters of the bladder neck and urethra, resulting in total loss of retentive ability.

Inflammation: Redness or swelling caused by injury or infection.

Informed Consent: Permission to proceed given by a patient after being fully informed of the purposes and potential consequences of a medical procedure.

Intensity Modulated Radiation Therapy (IMRT): The most recent state-of-the-art, computer-aided technique for delivering higher doses of radiation more accurately than either conventional External Beam Radiation or Conformal Radiation. The most advanced form of IMRT is Dynamic Adaptive Radiotherapy (DART).

Intermittent Androgen Deprivation (IAD): A temporary discontinuation of hormonal therapy that allows for a return to natural testosterone production in order to spare the patient from symptoms associated with androgen deprivation. Also referred to as Intermittent Hormonal Therapy (IHT).

Intravenous Pyelogram (IVP): A test that utilizes the injection of a special dye to check for injury or the spread of cancer to the kidneys and bladder.

Investigational: A drug or procedure allowed by the FDA for use in clinical trails, but not necessarily reimbursed.

Isodose Line: A line or two-dimensional shape that circumscribes an area receiving a radiation dose greater than or equal to a specified amount.

Laparoscopic Lymphadenectomy: The removal of pelvic lymph nodes with a laparoscope via four small incisions in the lower abdomen.

LH (Luteinizing Hormone): A chemical signal originating in the pituitary gland that causes the testes to make testosterone.

LHRH Analogs (or LHRH Agonists): Synthetic compounds that are chemically similar to Luteinizing Hormone Releasing Hormone (LHRH), used to suppress testicular production of testosterone. The most commonly prescribed LHRH analogs are Lupron® and Zoldex® Eligard® and Trelstar®. See also Luteinizing Hormone-Releasing Hormone (LHRH).

LHRH Antagonist: A chemical agent that blocks the LHRH receptor without the testosterone surge associated with

LHRH analogs. LHRH antagonists include Abarelix (Plenaxis®).

Linear Accelerator: A high energy x-ray machine generating radiation fields for external beam radiation therapy. These machines are typically mounted with a collimator (or multileaf collimator) in a gantry that rotates vertically around the patient being treated.

Localized Prostate Cancer: Cancer that is confined to the prostate gland, and therefore, considered curable.

Luteinizing Hormone-Releasing Hormone (LHRH): A chemical signal originating in the hypothalamus that causes the pituitary to make LH, which in turn stimulates the testicles to make testosterone.

Lymphadenectomy: The removal and examination of lymph nodes to precisely diagnose and stage cancer. See also Laparascopic Lymphadenectomy.

Lymph Node: A small, bean-shaped mass of tissue located throughout the body along the vessels of the lymphatic system. The lymph nodes filter out bacteria and other toxins, as well as cancer cells.

Magnetic Resonance Imaging (MRI): A painless, non-invasive technique using strong magnetic fields to produce detailed images of internal body structures. An MRI scan usually takes about 45 minutes per site.

Malignancy: A tumorous growth of cancer cells.

Malignant: Having the invasive and metastatic properties of cancer. Tending to become progressively worse and to result in death.

Margin: See Surgical Margin.

Metalloprotease Inhibitors: Drugs used to suppress the body's production of certain enzymes.

Metastasis: The spread of cancer, by way of the blood stream or lymphatic system, beyond the boundaries of the organ or structure where the cancer originated. Metastases is the plural. Metastatic refers to the characteristics associated with cancer that has spread or a secondary tumor.

Metastatic Work-Up: A group of tests, including bone scans, x-rays, and blood tests, to ascertain whether cancer has metastasized.

Monoclonal Antibody (mAb): An antibody that is directed against one specific protein (antigen).

Morbidity: Unhealthy consequences and complications resulting from treatment.

MRI: See Magnetic Resonance Imaging.

Nadir: The lowest point. Doctors sometimes use this as a verb to describe return of cancer or treatment failure. The PSA nadir refers to a minimum PSA value that should be maintained after treatment if the cancer has been successfully eradicated.

Necrosis: Death of cells or tissues caused by disease or injury.

Neoadjuvant: The use of a different type of therapy before primary, curative treatment. For example, neoadjuvant Androgen Deprivation Therapy is often used prior to radiation therapy or radical surgery, with the intent of improving the effectiveness of the primary treatment by reducing the size of the tumor and/or prostate gland.

Nerve-sparing: A procedure used during radical prostatectomy in which the surgeon attempts to save the nerves (neurovascular bundles) that allow for normal sexual functions.

Neurovascular Bundles: Strands of interwoven nerves and veins that run down the side of the prostate. The bundles contain microscopic nerves that are essential for erection; they also contain arteries and veins. Cutting the nerves in the bundles during surgery, or otherwise harming them in another procedure, usually renders the patient impotent.

Nocturia: Getting up at night to urinate.

Non-invasive: Not involving any incision in the body.

Oncogenes: Genes associated with tumor growth.

Oncology: The branch of medical science dealing with tumors. A medical oncologist is a specialist in the study of cancerous tumors.

Organ-confined Disease (OCD): Prostate cancer that is confined to the prostate gland, as indicated clinically or pathologically.

Orchiectomy: A simple operation that involves surgical removal of the testicles, which produce most of the body's testosterone.

Osteoporosis: A decrease in bone mass and density causing fragility and porosity.

Overstaging: An assessment of an overly high clinical stage at initial diagnosis.

Palliative: Affording symptomatic pain relieve but not cure or remission.

Palpable: Capable of being felt when examined by touch or manipulation.

PAP: See Prostatic Acid Phosphatase.

Pathologist: A doctor who specializes in the examination of cells and tissues removed from the body.

PBRT: See Proton Beam Radiation Therapy.

Perineum: The area of the body between the anus and scrotum. A perineal procedure uses this area as the point of entry into the body.

Perineural Invasion: Describing cancer, which has spread from the prostate to the nerve bundles.

Periprostatic: Relating to the soft tissues immediately proximate to the prostate gland.

Photon: The quantum of electromagnetic energy, described as having zero mass and no electric charge. X-rays are high energy photons.

Placebo: A sugar pill often taken by participants in a medical study. Patients taking a placebo are compared to patients taking actual medications.

Ploidy Analysis: A pathological analysis to determine the number of sets of chromosomes in a cell.

Proctitis: Inflammation of the rectum.

Prognosis: A forecast of the course of a disease and future prospects of the patient.

Progression: A change in the status of the cancer indicating the condition has progressed and worsened.

Pro-oxidant: A term to describe substances that aid in oxidation.

ProstaScint® Scan: An imaging technique sometimes used determine whether or not cancer has spread to distant sites by using monoclonal antibodies.

Prostate Capsule: It was once thought that the prostate gland was surrounded by a clearly identifiable capsule, but pathological studies have shown there is no capsule as such. The gland exists within a fat plane.

Prostatectomy: The surgical removal of part or all of the prostate gland.

Prostate Specific Antigen (PSA): A blood test that measures a substance manufactured solely by prostate gland cells. An elevated reading indicates an abnormal condition of the prostate gland, either benign or malignant. It is presently the most sensitive tumor marker for the identification and monitoring of prostate cancer.

Prostatic Acid Phosphatase (PAP): An enzyme produced by the prostate that is elevated (3.0 or higher) in many patients when prostate cancer has spread beyond the prostate.

Prostatitis: An infection or inflammation of the prostate gland that is treatable with medications.

Proton Beam Radiation Therapy (PBRT): A form of radiation therapy that utilizes protons as the source of energy (as opposed to X-rays or neutrons).

PSA: See Prostate Specific Antigen.

PSA Bounce (or PSA Bump): A rise in PSA level after first having a reduction in PSA after radiation therapy.

PSA Nadir: The lowest PSA value after a particular treatment.

PSA Velocity (PSAV): The rate of increase of the PSA level, expressed as nanograms per milliliter per year.

Radiation Therapy (RT): The use of high energy rays to kill cancer cells and malignant tissue.

Radiation Urethritis: Inflammation of the urethra caused by radiation therapy.

Radical Prostatectomy: An operation to remove the entire prostate gland and seminal vesicles.

Radiosensitivity: The degree to which a type of cancer responds to radiation therapy.

RBA or Relative Biological Effectiveness: A scale used to compare the intensity of radiation associated with various atomic particles.

Receptor: A cellular docking site that interacts with a specific protein or enzyme (called a ligand). The interaction typically leads to the synthesis of other substances such as proteins, hormones or enzymes.

Recurrence: Return of the cancer following remission or treatment intended as curative. Local recurrence indicates a return of the cancer at the site of origin. Distant recurrence indicates the appearance of one or more metastases of the disease.

Refractory: A term indicating that the cancer no longer responds to the current therapy.

Remission: Complete or partial disappearance of the signs and symptoms of the disease. The period during which a disease remains under control, without progressing. Even complete remission does not necessarily indicate cure.

Resection: The surgical removal of a part of an organ or structure.

Risk: The probability that a particular event will or will not happen.

RP: See Radical Prostatectomy.

RT: See Radiation Therapy.

Rx: The standard abbreviation for prescription.

Salvage Treatment: A medical term for "Plan B." It means a patient must undergo another form of treatment because the first therapy was not successful. Salvage therapy may incur a higher rate of side effects.

Saw Palmetto: A nutrient extracted from the saw palmetto shrub, which is considered by some to aid the body's immune system.

Seed Implantation (SI): A minimally invasive procedure by which radioactive seeds are implanted into the prostate gland to destroy cancer. Also referred to as seeding and brachytherapy.

Selenium: A non-metallic element thought to be beneficial as a nutrient; it is often included in multivitamin supplements.

Seminal Vesicles: Glands that, like the prostate, support male reproduction. Fluid secreted by these glands regulates the consistency of semen.

Side Effect: A reaction to a treatment or medication, usually referring to an undesirable effect.

Sphincter: A circular muscle which contracts to close an orifice. The urethral sphincter squeezes the urethra shut, providing urinary control.

Staging: The testing process by which the extent and severity of a known cancer is evaluated according to an established system of classification. It is used to help determine appropriate therapy. See TNM Staging and Whitmore-Jewett Staging.

Surgical Margin: The outer edge of the tissue removed during a radical prostatectomy. The surgical margin may be "negative," indicating that no cancer is present and a better prognosis, or "positive," indicating that not all of the cancer has been removed.

Systemic: Throughout the body and affecting the entire body.

T-Cell: An immune system cell or lymphocyte that directs an immune response to malignant or infected cells.

Testes: Two male reproductive glands located inside the scrotum. The testes are the primary sources for testosterone. Also called testicles.

Testosterone: A male sex hormone chiefly produced by the testicles.

Thrombotic: Causing or relating to blood clotting.

TNM Staging: The most widely used classification system for evaluating the extent of prostate cancer. TNM refers to tumor, nodes and metastases. See Staging.

Transrectal: Through the rectum.

Transurethral: Through the urethra.

Transrectal Ultrasonography: See Ultrasound.

Transurethral Resection of the Prostate (TURP): A surgical procedure to remove tissue obstructing the urethra. The technique involves the insertion of an instrument called a resectoscope into the penile urethra, and is intended to relieve obstruction of urine flow due to enlargement of the prostate.

Tumor: An excessive growth of cells that is caused by uncontrolled and disorderly cell replacement. Abnormal tissue growth may be benign or malignant. See also Benign, Malignant.

TURP: See Transurethral Resection of the Prostate.

Ultrasound (Transrectal Ultrasonography): A painless, non-invasive diagnostic imaging technique using sound waves to create an echo pattern that reveals the structure of organs and tissues. It does not use x-rays.

Understaging: An overly low assessment of clinical stage at diagnosis.

Urethra: The tube that carries urine from the bladder and semen from the prostate out of the body through the penis.

Urologist: A physician who specializes in the diagnosis and the medical and surgical treatment of problems in the urinary and male reproductive systems.

USPIO: This technology uses ultrasmall superparamagnetic iron oxide (USPIO) as an MRI contrast agent for the identification of cancer metastasis in lymph nodes.

Vasectomy: A surgical procedure to render a man sterile by cutting the vas deferens, thus eliminating the passage of sperm from the testes to the prostate.

Vasoactive: Causing the dilation or constriction of blood vessels.

Vesicle: A small sac containing fluid, as in seminal vesicles.

Whitmore-Jewett Staging: A classification system for evaluating the extent of prostate cancer. This system is less widely used for the designation of stage than is TNM staging.

X-rays: High energy radiation that can be used at low levels of intensity to make images of the body's internal structures, or at high intensity for radiation therapy.

APPENDIX E

THE WARNING SIGNS OF PROSTATE CANCER

There are often no warning signs of prostate cancer. In some cases the following symptoms may indicate the presence of the disease. However, please be aware that these symptoms may also be due to benign conditions of the prostate, or other conditions entirely unrelated to prostate cancer:

- ✔ Elevated or rising PSA
- ✔ Abnormal Digital Rectal Exam
- ✔ Blood in urine
- ✔ Pain or difficulty urinating
- ✔ Increased urge to urinate, especially at night
- ✔ Hesitant or intermittent urinary flow
- ✔ Pain or discomfort in area of prostate
- ✔ Unusual and unexplained weight loss
- ✔ Continual pain in lower back, hips or pelvis
- ✔ Increased voiding urgency
- ✔ Inability to urinate
- ✔ Trouble having or keeping an erection (erectile dysfunction)
- ✔ Weakness or numbness in the legs or feet

ABOUT THE AUTHORS

Michael J. Dattoli, M.D.

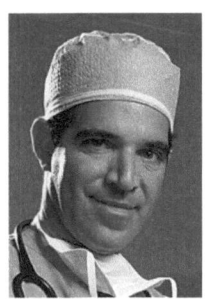
Michael J. Dattoli, MD, is a board-certified radiation oncologist with well over two decades of brachytherapy experience and has performed thousands of prostate implant procedures. He is considered the foremost pioneer in the field, optimizing brachytherapy designs to maximize tumor eradication and minimize symptoms. He has also been the leading trailblazer in the development of Dynamic Adaptive Radiotherapy (DART), utilizing all of the state-of-the-art modalities associated with 4-Dimensional Image-Guided Intensity Modulated Radiotherapy (3D-IMRT). Dr. Dattoli has successfully applied the same technologies to other forms of cancer, including breast, head and neck, GI, GYN, sarcomas and lung malignancies. He is a noted author and speaker in this complex field of medicine.

Dr. Dattoli attended the University of California at Berkeley and was the Valedictorian of his class at Vassar College; he earned his medical degree at Mount Sinai School of Medicine, Radiation Oncology at New York University Medical Center, then distinguished himself at Memorial Sloan-Kettering Cancer Center and New York Hospital-Cornell University Medical Center, as the Special Fellow in Brachytherapy. He was appointed Associate Professor in Brachytherapy and Radiation Oncology at Memorial Sloan- Kettering Cancer Center in New York and at New York Hospital-Cornell University Medical Center prior to relocating to Florida.

Dr. Dattoli also serves on multiple journal editorial review boards. Government appointments include "The Prostate Cancer Task Force" in Florida and consultant to the "Washington Oncology Roundtable Advisory Committee". He was selected by the International Association of Oncologists as a Leading Physician of the World and top Brachytherapist.

Michael M. Kaminski, M.D.

Joseph M. Kaminski, MD, previously Senior Medical Staff at the National Cancer Institute at the National Institutes of Health, is a board certified Radiation Oncologist who is internationally known for his work in accelerating the development of cancer therapeutics including normal tissue radioprotectors/mitigators, imaging techniques, and important interventional devices.

Dr. Kaminski has authored more than 70 publications in peer reviewed journals and has served on multiple journal editorial boards. He has also held positions as a Lead Medical Officer at the Food and Drug Administration and a medical officer at the National Institutes of Allergy and Infectious Diseases. He graduated with highest honors from Georgia Institute of Technology, one of the nation's top bioengineering universities, and completed medical school at the Medical College of Georgia.

Dr. Kaminski was a resident in Nuclear Medicine and Radiation Oncology at Vanderbilt University Medical Center (Nashville, TN), and also in Radiation Oncology at the prestigious Fox Chase Cancer Center (Philadelphia, PA). He joined the Dattoli team after working at Georgia Regents University where he served as the Co-Leader of the Neurological Oncology Multidisciplinary Program for the Cancer Center and the Director of Genitourinary (e.g., prostate), Gastrointestinal, and Central Nervous System Radiation Programs.

THE DATTOLI CANCER FOUNDATION MISSION

The Dattoli Cancer Foundation, sponsor of the Prostate Cancer Resource Network, is a 501(c)(3), tax-exempt charitable organization, whose mission is

- to raise awareness of the wide-spread incidence of Prostate Cancer and the need for early and annual screenings;

- to provide information and support to men newly diagnosed with Prostate Cancer as well as to those with recurrent Prostate Cancer, and

- to foster research into better diagnostic tools and treatment options for Prostate Cancer.

Gifts to the Dattoli Foundation make possible publications like this one, and are welcomed anytime. A copy of the official registration and financial information may be obtained from the Division of Consumer Services by calling toll-free (800-435-7352) within the state. Registration does not imply endorsement, approval or recommendations by the state.

Dattoli Cancer Foundation
2803 Fruitville Road
Sarasota, FL 34237
941/365-5599
800/915-1001
fax: 941/332-2317
www.dattolifoundation.org

ORDER MORE BOOKLETS IN THE SERIES

This *Prostate Cancer Essentials for Survival* booklet was published by the Datolli Cancer Foundation. For a complete list of booklets in the series and ordering information, please visit the Dattoli Cancer Center Book Shelf at dattoli.com/book-shelf. Current titles include::

- ✔ Coping with Prostate Cancer Recurrence
- ✔ Conquering Prostate Cancer with DART and Brachytherapy
- ✔ The Dattoli Prostate Cancer Challenge: Evaluating All Your Treatment Options
- ✔ The Facts: Comparing Prosate Cancer Treatment Options
- ✔ Dynamic Adaptive Radiotherapy
- ✔ Interpreting Your PSA Results: And Related Prostate Cancer Lab Tests
- ✔ Dosimetry and Prostate Cancer Radiotherapy
- ✔ Advanced Imaging for Prostate Cancer: A Primer on 3D Color-Flow Power Doppler Ultrasound, Multiparametric MRI and CT Fusion Techniques
- ✔ Image-Guided Prostate Biopsy: When, Why and What to Expect
- ✔ Hormonal Therapy for Prostate Cancer: The Benefits and Risks
- ✔ Lymph Node Positive Prostate Cancer: Advanced Diagnostics and Treatment
- ✔ The Dattoli Blue Ribbon Prostate Cancer Solution: How to Survive and Thrive Without Surgery

www.ingramcontent.com/pod-product-compliance
Lightning Source LLC
Chambersburg PA
CBHW040237220526
45473CB00001B/275